# Finding Grace in Caregiving

# Finding Grace in Caregiving

BRADLEY C. HANSON

CASCADE *Books* • Eugene, Oregon

FINDING GRACE IN CAREGIVING

Copyright © 2021 Bradley C. Hanson. All rights reserved. Except for brief quotations in critical publications or reviews, no part of this book may be reproduced in any manner without prior written permission from the publisher. Write: Permissions, Wipf and Stock Publishers, 199 W. 8th Ave., Suite 3, Eugene, OR 97401.

Cascade Books
An Imprint of Wipf and Stock Publishers
199 W. 8th Ave., Suite 3
Eugene, OR 97401

www.wipfandstock.com

PAPERBACK ISBN: 978-1-7252-7405-1
HARDCOVER ISBN: 978-1-7252-7406-8
EBOOK ISBN: 978-1-7252-7407-5

*Cataloguing-in-Publication data:*

Names: Hanson, Bradley C., author.

Title: Finding grace in caregiving / Bradley C. Hanson.

Description: Eugene, OR: Cascade Books, 2021.

Identifiers: ISBN 978-1-7252-7405-1 (paperback) | ISBN 978-1-7252-7406-8 (hardcover) | ISBN 978-1-7252-7407-5 (ebook)

Subjects: LCSH: Christian caregiving. | Caring—Religious aspects—Christianity. | Alzheimer's disease and dementia.

Classification: BV4509.5 .H50 2021 (print) | BV4509.5 (ebook)

# Table of Contents

1. A Forthright Family Conversation  1
2. Our Entry into Extended Caregiving  6
3. Love  23
4. Joy  32
5. Peace  49
6. Patience  86
7. Kindness  99
8. Goodness  121
9. Faithfulness  125
10. Gentleness  135
11. Relationships and Spiritual Practices in Caregiving  142

CHAPTER ONE

# A Forthright Family Conversation

*Kim Hanson to Brad Hanson, Carter Hanson, Michelle Hanson, Julie Hanson-Perez, Monchy Perez, Pamela Liu, October 1, 2017*

>Hi all. I have been slowly talking to Bryce about Mom. He wrote this in his third grade school journal today: "I'm worried about Grandma with her Alzheimers."
>Kim

*Bradley Hanson to Kim, Pam, Carter, Michelle, Julie, Monchy, October 2, 2017*

>Kim,
>
>Thanks for talking with Bryce about Mom. We're only part way on this journey, so it's good to clue in Bryce about her now. She is still the extremely kind, gentle woman we've known all along, but her short-term memory is weak and also some of her longer-term memories are not there for her now.
>
>Love,
>
>Dad

*Julie to Brad, Kim, Pam, Monchy, Carter, Michelle, October 2, 2017*

>Thanks for sharing Bryce's journal entry, Kim. I can imagine it would be rather difficult to talk with him about this.
>
>I wanted to let you all know how it went when I stayed with Mom the weekend of September 22. There were a few things that

stood out for me. One was just how she struggles to find words as she talks. She gets frustrated when that happens and makes comments about her brain not working right.

We had a nice time looking through the book of photos and memories that Dad put together for Mom's seventieth birthday. She pulled it out when I asked her a question about her work at the Area I Agency on Agency [a program of the Federal Department of Elder Affairs] because she thought it might help her answer my question (and it did).

It seems like having a regular routine is helpful in terms of knowing what to do and when. She knows when lunch, afternoon tea, afternoon walk, dinner, and watching TV all normally happen. I think Mom and Dad must often have had potatoes for dinner because it really seemed to confuse her when I didn't want one. She must have asked me twenty times within about seven minutes if I wanted a potato.

She talked quite a bit about when she was growing up and there are a couple of stories that she tells again and again. She has a difficult time figuring out relationships. She asked me a couple times if I knew her brother and sisters. Then she would say that her sister Anne was a nice lady or a nice girl but it was like she was talking about someone she didn't really know very well.

There were two moments that were particularly sad for me. One was when we were sitting out on the deck and she asked me about my parents. I asked her what she meant and she wondered where my parents lived when I was growing up. I said, "You're my mom, so here in Decorah." She said, "Oh, I didn't think about that."

The other sad moment was the following day when she gave me a hug and told me she was glad I was her cousin.

I was glad to have the opportunity to spend the weekend with her. It was a relaxing time and we had some nice talks and enjoyed our walks. I have an even greater appreciation for Dad's patience when she asks the same question multiple times (which happened a lot). I also have a great admiration for Mom and how she continues to be such a positive and caring person in spite of what she's going through.

Love to you all,

Julie

# A Forthright Family Conversation

*Brad to Julie, et al., October 2, 2017*

> Thanks for sharing your thoughts and observations about Mom from your weekend alone with her.
>
> From what I've read about Alzheimer's Disease, I gather that the person's cognitive memory declines and eventually is lost altogether; the person's emotional memory lasts longer. For example, I spoke recently with a man who is in his early sixties. His mother has Alzheimer's and his dad has Parkinson's. Both are in a nursing home now, in separate rooms. This man said that his mother does not speak his name, and it's been two months since she said, "You're my son." Yet she still will accept his help and intervention (over that of her husband or nursing home staff), if she is troubled or disturbed about something. So emotionally, she still has a special connection with her son.
>
> Julie, Mom's calling you her cousin seems consistent with this disconnect between cognitive memory and emotional memory. In Mom's case, when reminded or corrected, she immediately recognizes that you're her daughter, but she can't always make that cognitive connection on her own.
>
> Love to all,
>
> Dad/Brad

About a month earlier, I had sent this update on Marion in an email to our three kids—Julie, Carter, Kim—and their spouses.

*Brad to Julie, Carter, Kim, Monchy, Michelle, Pam, August 23, 2017*

> I think Mom has moved into the middle stage of Alzheimer's Disease. The Alzheimer's Association website, which reflects accepted medical opinion on the disease, divides the progression of Alzheimer's into three stages: mild (early stage), moderate (middle stage), and severe (late stage). We've known that Mom has been in the mild, early stage for quite a long time. That may be because of her own knowledge and experience with Alzheimer's people through her work with the Area Agency on Agency, from which she retired in 1996. Mom herself was the one who pressed to have herself examined for onset of dementia at the Mayo Clinic already, I think, in 2003 and again probably two years later and, then again in 2008 when she was diagnosed with mild cognitive deficit (often a preliminary to Alzheimer's) and then Alzheimer's Disease in

2010. I've always admired her tremendous courage and openness in dealing with this, in contrast to many who persistently deny it.

The advance of the disease has occurred gradually. Her ability to express herself in words has declined little by little over the last several years, but her difficulty with this has grown to the point that it's more frequent and more obvious. Another indication has been a decline in her ability to drive safely and find her destination and return home. Up until late May Mom was driving some, although not a lot. But as you can appreciate, the ability to drive is a huge marker of personal independence, so it's tough to give up. I decided that it would be mutually beneficial for Carter's family and for Mom and me that we give our 2004 Toyota to Carter and Michelle on their return from Germany. Although Mom said that would be OK, at times she resisted that step. But it happened. In July after we were down to one car, one time (I don't recall where I was) she drove down to Fareway to buy a few groceries, but when she got there, she couldn't remember what she was supposed to get, so she came home again.

I've attached information from the Alzheimer's Association website describing the three stages and also their info about caregiving during each stage. We've been through the easy, first stage, but now we're moving into the second stage. Of course, I intend to be the primary caregiver for Mom. But I cannot continue to do that entirely by myself. It is critical for me to find relief and get away now and then. I think it's too early yet to be using adult daycare opportunities, but it's realistic to expect that will become a staple at some point. For now I'm scheduled to go on a two-day private retreat September 22 to 24, a few miles east of La Crosse. Julie has graciously agreed to be here with Mom during that time. It's not likely that Mom would do anything crazy while alone in the house, but there might be an instance in which she would leave a kitchen stove burner on and a housefire could result.

Carter and Kim, since you're much farther away than Julie, any relief that you might give would most likely have to be arranged to fit your schedule. For now, and the near term, I expect that my getting away twice a year may be enough. I would appreciate, though, the willingness of all of you to participate in the planning for Mom's care.

We both have long-term care insurance, so when entrance into a care facility becomes necessary (in the third stage, I suppose), we should be able to handle the expense. But even prior to that, it may be prudent to hire some help to assist us at home. Another option is to enter an assisted living facility (there are three in

## A Forthright Family Conversation

Decorah) where we would have our own apartment, but get meals and some help with cleaning and laundry. We'll just have to make these judgments as we go along, and I'd like to involve Mom in making those judgments as much as is possible for her. Mom and I also ask for your support in prayer. She is an incredibly kind, gentle person. I don't think I've ever heard a mean word come from her mouth. I have been amazingly blessed by sharing these fifty-five years with her.

By the way, Mom and I are dropping out of our four-couple game group that has met monthly since sometime in the early 1970s. Laursens are the only remaining original members. It's become too hard for Mom to participate in whatever board game or card game the host couple chooses. I suggested dropping out a year ago, but Mom didn't want to do that. When I suggested it again several weeks ago, she agreed. We'll meet for the final time this Saturday, August 26, for dinner at the home of John and Lindy Moeller (this was John's idea). It's a happy coincidence that Saturday will be our fifty-fifth wedding anniversary.

Love to all,

Dad/Brad

CHAPTER TWO

# Our Entry into Extended Caregiving

LIKE A GREAT MANY other people, my first substantial engagement with caring for someone unable to provide for themselves came when our first child, Julie, was born. She was totally dependent upon Marion and me. She could not obtain her own nourishment or keep herself warm and clean. Caring for an infant may not be what first comes to mind when we speak of "caregiving," because that term often has a narrower reference. As Wikipedia says, "A caregiver or carer is an unpaid or paid member of a person's social network who helps them with activities of daily living. Caregiving is most commonly used to address impairments related to old age, disability, a disease, or a mental disorder." It is good to recognize, though, that the essential dynamics of caregiving—providing for the needs of someone unable to care adequately for themselves—are present more broadly in human experience. The most common experience of caregiving is parenting a young child. Indeed, *The Merriam-Webster Dictionary* gives this broader definition: "Caregiving is the activity or profession of regularly looking after a child or a sick, elderly, or disabled person." The basic point is that there are diverse circumstances that call for caregiving, for helping someone meet their basic needs for life and well-being.

If we are not a professional caregiver, our first significant personal encounter with what we usually label "caregiving" is most commonly with an older family member and often involves experience with dementia. In my own case, I had very little involvement in caregiving for my two elderly grandmothers, because during that time I was mostly away at college. I recall that my recently widowed maternal grandmother gave up her apartment and moved in with one of my aunts until Grandma's death. My

## Our Entry into Extended Caregiving

paternal grandmother—in her early nineties—lived independently until shortly before her death.

My own experience with caregiving someone elderly began and gradually increased as my parents advanced into their eighties. Mom and Dad lived in their own home three hours away from us. About every four to six weeks I alone or Marion and I would drive to their house and stay one or two nights. Mostly we were just monitoring their situation. Dad had arranged for help with mowing and snow removal, and they were able to do their own simple shopping, meal preparation, and laundry. However, when Mom was in her early eighties, Marion alerted me to Mom's memory deficiency. One time Marion and I met them for lunch at a McDonald's in a town that was midway between our homes. Afterward Marion pointed out that going to their car to return home, Mom had first started to get in the rear seat before Dad corrected her. This and a couple of other incidents during our lunchtime conversation suggested memory deficiency to Marion.

I observed Mom's dementia up close after Dad and she came to live with us at the end of June in 1994. At that point Dad was ninety-one and Mom was eighty-seven, and their ability to manage on their own was compromised. Her home physician provided us with a detailed description of her medical condition that included the observation that she had some memory loss due to some small strokes. Dad had quite good health and mobility for his age. Mom and Dad took over our main floor bedroom, the adjoining study for their sitting room, and a bathroom, while downstairs Marion and I had our bedroom that looked out onto our wooded backyard, bathroom, and a sitting room with a separate exit door. We shared the kitchen, living-dining room, and laundry room on the main floor. On weekdays Marion and I were generally out of the house at work before Mom and Dad got up, but we had the evening meal together. Marion's burden of caregiving greatly increased four months after their arrival, when I had major surgery for colon cancer in late October of that same year and soon began a year of weekly chemotherapy infusions. Now Marion was also caregiving me.

Mom and Dad managed quite well in their new situation. They got their own breakfast and lunch, and took their dog (oh, yes, they always had a dog) out for short walks. The most obvious indication of Mom's memory loss was the repeated times she asked Dad what day it was. What was so remarkable to me was that Dad never raised his voice in answering her.

He was extraordinarily patient with her. Every time I recall his patience, I choke up with admiration and gratitude for my dad.

However, over their fifteen months with us, their gradually increasing fragility and liability of falling finally led me to suggest to Dad that it was time to move to a nursing home in our town. Without protest, he agreed. At the nursing home they shared a room, and Marion and I visited them every day that we were in town. After a little more than a year, Dad was diagnosed with advanced colon cancer and died a few weeks later. Soon Mom moved to a private room. Her memory continued to gradually decline, but she always recognized Marion or me instantly. Her face always lit up with a smile when she saw us coming to see her. Early one morning a major stroke ended her life.

Looking back upon this time of caregiving for my parents, I am deeply grateful for the experience. My admiration for them grew greatly. Their profound trust, commitment, love, and support for each other let me see the fruit of a long, devoted marriage. I received much more than I gave. An occasional visit with them during these last years of their lives would not have been nearly so rewarding for me, and would have given them far less security. A bonus blessing for me was seeing the extraordinary kindness and patience of Marion in caring for my parents as well as for me in my recovery from colon cancer.

All of us approach this matter of caregiving with our own personal and family experience of caregiving. Many of us with children have already done extensive caregiving, although we may not have seen the connections between childcare and caregiving someone who is ill or infirm. Those who care for a person with special needs are especially aware of what it takes to do loving care for the long haul.

## Caregiving Marion

The journey with caregiving Marion that I and our three children have experienced has been in some respects atypical, because of Marion's prior work experience with individuals and families doing caregiving through her job with our regional Area Agency on Aging. As program coordinator for about twenty-five programs, ordinarily working directly with those doing caregiving at home would have been the responsibility of someone else under Marion's supervision, but after progress in this area lagged at her agency, she took over that task herself.

## Our Entry into Extended Caregiving

As part of her responsibility for home caregiving, Marion gave special emphasis to the major need for caregiving persons with dementia. She organized an Alzheimer's support group in each of her five counties, and visited many families affected by Alzheimer's and other conditions causing dementia. Characteristically, she also read deeply and attended conferences on these topics. As a result, Marion had a considerable understanding of dementia and especially Alzheimer's disease when in early 1996 at the age of fifty-six she retired, in order to devote her full attention to a three-year program for becoming a spiritual director.

Several years later I was surprised when she arranged to have an April 2003 examination of herself by a neurologist at Mayo Clinic in Rochester, Minnesota. I accompanied her, of course, but I had not noticed any major memory lapses. Following the exam, the neurologist wrote, "Her MRI of the brain with the Jack protocol was unremarkable. Her four-hour neuropsychometric testing did not show any significant cognitive deficits and was suggestive that depression could be the etiology of her complaints of cognitive inefficiency."

The neurologist referred her to a Mayo psychiatrist, whose clinical notes from that same day said:

> She has identified two issues.
>
> 1. Memory.
>
> She feels that for the past one year she has been having some difficulties such as misplacing things, sometimes not knowing the day, forgetting appointments, at times she gets surprised when guests arrive to her house forgetting that she had arranged an appointment with them. She also tends to forget things that are recent events at times. If her beloved ones call her and talk to her about an item, she is able to remember most of it by and large. She does not have any problem with sense of direction. She is able to understand and express herself very well. However, she has noticed that she is having some difficulty with her reading comprehension and it is not as sharp as it used to be.
>
> 2. Depression
>
> She reports that she tends to have mild depression particularly during winter time.

Marion followed the recommendation of these Mayo doctors that she undergo cognitive behavioral therapy and began meeting with a local psychologist. Her personal notes preparatory for one such meeting from November 2004 reveal her detailed awareness of a variety of memory deficits:

> Don't remember if took pills or dusted a piece of furniture. Can't recall conversations—may remember one thing, but not the reasons, the sequences, the problems, the solutions, within same day.
> Can't recall names; can see faces in mind.
> Conversation difficult—words don't come out in right order or I can't say what I'm thinking. Can't think of words to convey it.
> Don't remember activities, seeing someone.
> Have difficulty remembering date month—season.
> Concentration difficult in conversations—don't really listen.
> Walk down the street, have to really think about what direction to turn, where something is.
> Very little motivation.

Marion's second visit with the Mayo neurologist and psychiatrist in 2005 produced no significant change, but at her third visit in 2008 the neurologist told us that her condition was now *mild cognitive impairment*. This is the medical term for a condition with symptoms more severe than typical aging, but not severe enough to be considered dementia. Not everyone with mild cognitive impairment goes on to dementia; some stay at this stage and others even return to normal cognition.[1]

In 2010, we were not surprised when the neurologist now called it Alzheimer's disease. He said that while people often comment that an autopsy is the only sure way to identify Alzheimer's, "We get it right 97 percent of the time." Because throughout our conversation he had been looking only at me, I asked him to speak not just to me, but to both of us. The fact that his behavior treated her as though she were already not present hurt and angered me. She is a person who matters.

Everyone's journey with dementia has both unique and common aspects. While being *this* individual with *this particular* family history is unique, there are some features of the dementia journey that are broadly shared. One common aspect is the process of recognizing and admitting that I or a loved one has a disease that causes dementia.

---

1. Ronald C. Petersen, medical ed., *Mayo Clinic on Alzheimer's Disease* (Rochester, MN: Mayo Clinic, 2013), 102.

OUR ENTRY INTO EXTENDED CAREGIVING

## Recognizing and Acknowledging Dementia

A highly unusual feature of my own family's experience with dementia is that Marion, the affected person herself, was the one who carefully monitored herself for memory loss and pressed repeatedly to be examined for signs of dementia. It is far more common that the one developing dementia is slow to recognize, much less admit, possible signs of dementia. Usually, it is only in retrospect that early indications are understood by others and even later by the one with dementia.

Typical is the experience of this husband, a medical doctor that I'll identify as C, with whom I spoke in 2017. C tells how early signs of his wife's memory loss were ignored or explained away:

> We've been married fifty-nine years, and we've had a great marriage. Then my situation changed. Two or three years ago, for example, she wanted to learn about the computer. Each time we tried, it was as though she was there for the first time. I'd get very angry. I'd leave, throwing up my hands. And she'd leave the same.
>
> It became more obvious that something was wrong. So I have become a caretaker, basically. In the sense that she takes care of all her bodily needs. I help her with the wash and folding. I do all the cooking. But the basic needs, she still takes care on her own.
>
> Brad: So you've become the household manager?
>
> Yah, and that meets with some sort of objections [chuckle].
> I've come to realize that she *really* had some medical problems already in 2015 at Christmas: sending two checks to the same son-in-law, and wrapping presents that could have been better wrapped by a kindergartner. Really raised some flags.

While many people equate dementia with Alzheimer's disease, actually dementia can result from a considerable number of medical conditions including Parkinson's disease, dementia with Lewy bodies, and vascular disorders such as high blood pressure that triggers a series of small strokes in the brain that produce areas of dead tissue called infarcts. The Mayo Clinic's book on Alzheimer's disease says, "Many people think of dementia as a disease. In fact, dementia is a syndrome, which means it's a collection of signs and symptoms caused by a disease."[2] The book goes on to say that memory loss is a common symptom of dementia, but memory

---
2. Peterson, ed., *Mayo Clinic on Alzheimer's Disease*, 38.

loss alone does not mean one has dementia. Dementia involves difficulty with memory loss and at least one other cognitive function. Johns Hopkins authors Nancy Mace and Peter Rabins say that while Alzheimer's is the most common cause of memory loss among older people, about one-third of older people suffer from dementia caused by a different disease.[3]

Dementia is caused by quite a few medical conditions, but the early signs of that condition may not be memory lapses. For instance, the wife of a man who received a doctor's diagnosis of Parkinson's disease in fall of 2001 recalls that the first indications that something was wrong were not obvious memory problems.

> At first he couldn't button his shirt—those tiny buttons, tie his necktie. Shoe strings were a problem, how to tie a necktie. Well, *I* didn't know how to tie a necktie. So you just go to sport shirts and Velcro shoes. Just getting in and out of a car. Early on, he fell a lot, early on.
>
> I don't think I noticed them during that last year he worked—2000–2001. His writing was getting really tiny, you could hardly read it. He would get very tired, and he had a little tremor in his left foot, but he could hide that under his desk at work and otherwise he was standing. And that last year, he complained about being tired. By the end of a heavy work day, he would be just exhausted. But those were the only things we noticed.
>
> But we didn't think too much of it until after the diagnosis, when you look back. But I didn't think, "Oh you're tired, so you've got Parkinson's." But as far as *remembering* things, I didn't notice anything at all.

Johns Hopkins School of Medicine authors Nancy Mace and Peter Rabins say:

> Usually the symptoms of dementia appear gradually. Sometimes the afflicted person may be the first to notice something wrong . . .
>
> People respond to their problems in different ways. Some people become skillful at concealing the difficulty. Some keep lists to jog their memory. Some vehemently deny that anything is wrong or blame their problems on others. Some people become depressed or irritable when they realize that their memory is failing. Others remain outwardly cheerful. Usually, the person who has mild to moderate dementia is able to continue to do most of

---

3. Nancy L. Mace and Peter V. Rabins, *The 36-Hour Day: A Family Guide to Caring for People Who Have Alzheimer's Disease, Related Dementias, and Memory Loss* (New York: Grand Central Life & Style), 10.

## Our Entry into Extended Caregiving

the things he has always done. Like a person with any other disease, he is able to participate in his treatment, family decisions, and planning for the future.[4]

As the condition worsens, two adjustments often made when financially feasible, are physical changes to the home living space and hiring outside help to assist with care. Physical changes to home living space are particularly critical with Parkinson's, since balance becomes an increasing problem. As one wife commented, "Falling, rigidity were just coming fast for him. Yah, we took quite a few tumbles. That's why we did the ramp [into the house]. Balance is a big thing with Parkinson's."

Another wife related several night-time incidents in which her husband with Parkinson's got up, and then got stuck somewhere in the house and could not return to bed.

> Before I remodeled the bathroom, . . . he got out of bed and needed to go to the bathroom and he got stuck [in the bathroom] and the wheel chair got jammed. Then I got [a neighbor man] over and he couldn't get him up, and then our daughter-in-law came and she couldn't get him up. And she just hopped up on the counter and onto the other side. And that was just hysterical.
>
> Another time I woke up in the middle of the night and he was not in bed, and so I looked around the house and went into every room, and checked every outside door and they were all locked, and I could not see him any place. I checked again more slowly, and I found him in a very small space in the spare bedroom. There he was on the floor with a pillow under his head. And he had gone in there by himself. He hadn't fallen. He had done it deliberately. And I couldn't get him up. So I called 911 and had EMTs come and help.
>
> And then another time, I woke up in the middle of the night, and he was not in bed. It was very easy to find him that time. He had gone into the living room to watch TV and tipped over in the wheelchair. But both the wheelchair and he were lying on the floor and [he was] watching TV.
>
> He had a pneumonia about two years before he passed away and went to a nursing home . . . at the time, for a month. And, of course, he just didn't like it. While he was there, I made a complete remodeling of the bathroom, completely gutted it, and made it accessible to a wheelchair. So I paid eleven hundred dollars, so he could come home. So I think he had a very good year at home.

---

4. Mace and Rabins, *The 36-Hour Day*, 10.

Another time I woke up in the morning and that was fine, and I came out to start some breakfast things while he was in the bathroom taking care of himself. When I came out here in the dining room, here was a pile of things two feet high or better of clothes and towels and shoes. When he came out, I said, "What is this about?" He said, "Well, I thought I would leave." *We* were not having problems. We were getting along fine. But apparently he wanted to travel. So I said, "Where were you going to go?" I tried his hometown? My family in Ohio? Visit his college in New Jersey? Nashville? Everything I could think of. Finally, he said, "I thought I'd go to Kansas City." And there was no reason to go to Kansas City. It was a total mystery. He had no particular connection with Kansas City. He had gone there once. Then in his wheelchair, he'd taken out shirts and socks, undershorts, towels from the bathroom. He was really ready to travel. It was getting a little scary, and unpredictable about what he might do.

As caregiving responsibilities increase, another adjustment a caregiver may make, if financially feasible and acceptable to the patient, is to hire someone to assist with household tasks and perhaps patient care for a few hours a week. As one wife, whose husband had Parkinson's, said:

The caretaker does the thinking for two people. You become the person who is the administrator, nursing person, the cook, the shopper, the baker—everything. This was the concern of my sister . . . whose husband was in a wheelchair and a walker. They got to a graduation in Wisconsin. She got there and discovered that she left all her dress clothes at home. She was hard on herself. "How could I do that?" I said, "You're going to find this more and more. You're doing everything for two people." You find out a different way to do it. You just have to adjust. You find out that you can become very creative, don't you? This doesn't work, or this is a problem, I've got to solve it, what do I have to do to make this easier? You become very inventive. I said, "I think I could become an inventor now."

And I got help in, and that was good. I had to have time to do my own business, my own doctor appointments and such. And I couldn't really leave him alone. I had to go do errands. I'd say, "I'm going downstairs for the laundry," and I wouldn't be even to the bottom of the steps and he would be calling, where was I? He just didn't like to be left alone either. So that's when I got help in, to help get him out of bed in the morning, showered, get breakfast, ready for going down for his nap again. If you have long-term care insurance, you just have to be sure that you have your ninety days in, within a certain time, even if you have them for only one hour a day with some of the insurances. I don't remember how long we had them. Anyway, I had them for several years.

I was fortunate. I have outside help, and I was fortunate to have our son here, and he said, "I'm ready to come at any time, day or night. I have a sweatshirt by my bed, and just call if you need help." He would fall in the middle of the night some nights. He'd actually crash like a tree. We have a few dents in the sheet rock. He just sprung the bi-fold closet drawers, and my brother had to take the whole thing apart. Dent in the car. But that's what it is.

Another wife whose husband had Parkinson's disease said that by the last five years of his life, she realized it was more unsafe for him to be alone, so she hired someone to do some household tasks. This allowed her time to run some errands with the confidence that her husband was safe.

While denial of a condition leading to memory loss is common, even someone who early on acknowledges having such a condition may resist a more extensive level of care. As one wife said of her husband with Parkinson's, "When he was first diagnosed, one of the first things he said was, 'I know what this path is, I know where this goes.' But when it comes right down to it, it becomes harder. And because of the dementia, he didn't really understand. It becomes harder. But it was just kind of crashing down. So entering a care facility is a difficult thing to do."

## Other Forms of Caregiving

Although caregiving happens often as care for the elderly, in fact, caregiving may happen in different forms and degrees throughout the human life cycle. *A caregiver does what is necessary for someone else's life and well-being when that person is not able to do it on his or her own.* Some persons are born with a condition that requires extensive lifelong care, and others from accident or combat suffer physical or psychological injury severe enough to require special care. But almost all parents are caregivers for their young children. As newborns and infants, we are totally dependent on adults for our nourishment and entire well-being; left on our own, we would die within a short time. As young children, we commonly rely upon parents or grandparents to provide food and clothing as well as protection and social support. Later as teenagers we usually draw upon varying forms of adult aid. So, there are different forms and degrees of giving and receiving care.

Furthermore, since we humans flourish only in community, we may provide caregiving not only for this or that individual person, but we may also provide *caregiving to a treasured community*. For most of us our primary community is our family, but in some cases, we also care deeply about certain other communities. As a college faculty member, I have observed strongly committed alumni devote precious time and resources to serving as a member of the board of regents. The well-being of every religious congregation also depends upon committed lay members who devote a significant portion of their time, energy, and treasure to the congregation. When I think of my own congregation, several persons immediately come to mind as exemplary in their high level of commitment to the congregation.

Passionate caregiving for a community is evident in the first-century letters of Paul the apostle. As a Christian missionary, Paul traveled widely under hazardous conditions in the ancient near East, preaching the gospel of Jesus Christ and establishing fledgling Christian congregations in many areas around the Mediterranean Sea. It may be difficult for us today to appreciate the depth of Paul's care for the Christian communities he had founded. While we might credit his deep caring to his being such a holy person, there were also very strong human factors that formed Paul's deep bonds with those communities. Central among these human factors were the enormous difficulties, obstacles, and hazards that Paul faced in carrying out his mission.

One measure of Paul's very strong human bond with his fledgling Christian communities is seen in the strenuousness of his travel in establishing and ministering to those communities. New Testament scholar Moyer Hubbard points out that travel in the ancient Mediterranean world had become more feasible by Paul's time because of the extensive road system that the Roman Empire constructed in its vast empire. Nevertheless, Hubbard says that travel was not only often dangerous, but also full of hardships. Danger came from bandits who made travel by land risky and from pirates and storms that threatened those on sailing ships. In addition to the dangers, travel at that time was arduous. He says, "When undertaking an overland journey, most people had little choice but to travel on foot. Horses were expensive and used mainly by the military and imperial couriers. Merchants and farmers transporting goods might use a cart drawn by a mule or a team of oxen. The wealthy elite could travel in grand style: wagons hauled by horses, carriages drawn by slaves, a huge entourage. Wheeled

## Our Entry into Extended Caregiving

transport, however, was not a realistic alternative for most."[5] This means that in founding Christian communities Paul often walked long distances.

For example, Acts 13:4–6 tells us about the beginning of Paul's first of three extensive missionary journeys, this one with his companion Barnabas:

> So, being sent out by the Holy Spirit, they went down to Seleucia; and from there they sailed to Cyprus. When they arrived at Salamis, they proclaimed the word of God in the synagogues of the Jews. And they had John also to assist them. When they had gone through the whole island as far as Paphos, they met a certain magician...

This tells us that after Paul and Barnabas were commissioned as missionaries by the church in Antioch of Syria, they went from Antioch to the nearby Mediterranean coastal town of Seleucia, from which they sailed to Salamis on the island of Cyprus, a distance of about 265 miles.

For an evangelist today this trip would be easy. One could fly from Antioch to Cyprus in about an hour flight time, pick up a rental car, and drive anywhere on the island in just a few hours. But Paul sailed to Cyprus on a boat that did not have the comfortable seating, toilet facilities, and food service we take for granted on a ferry boat today, much less the luxurious accommodations of a contemporary cruise ship. On his sailboat journey Paul would have been exposed to the sun and weather. Acts 13:6 tells us that after preaching at the city of Salamis in Cyprus, Paul and Barnabas "had gone through the whole island as far as Paphos" at the opposite end of the island. So it is very likely that Paul went from his starting point on Cyprus at the port town of Salamis to Nicosia, a major city toward the center of the island. This trip from Salamis to Nicosia, a distance of about forty-five miles, would have been on foot. The biblical phrase "a day's journey," which occurs in Luke 2:44 and John 3:4, is commonly understood to mean a journey around twenty miles on foot.[6] So Paul's travel from Salamis to Nicosia would have taken him a little more than two days of steady walking. Acts goes on to say, "When they had gone through the whole island as far as Paphos." This tells us that Paul and Barnabas traveled to the farthest point on the island. The straight, overland distance from their starting point on Cyprus to Paphos is about 100 miles, but Paul's indirect route would have

---

5. Moyer V. Hubbard, *Christianity in the Greco-Roman World* (Peabody, MA: Hendrickson, 2010), 119–20.

6. Hubbard, *Christianity in the Greco-Roman World*, 119–20.

required perhaps some short distance sailing, but also considerable walking. No doubt, Paul's travel on Cyprus was strenuous.

But Cyprus was just the beginning of Paul's first missionary journey. His next major stop according to Acts 13:13 was Perga in Pamphylia, which is located on the Mediterranean coast of modern Turkey. Getting there would have required sailing from Paphos on Cyprus to the Turkish coast, a distance of about 370 miles. Acts goes on to mention Paul's visits to several other cities in what is central Turkey today: Antioch in Pisidia (about 125 miles from the coast), Iconium of Pisidia, Lystra, and Derbe. Paul's travel to these cities would likely have been on foot, in good conditions walking twenty miles a day.

The rigor and danger of Paul's missionary travels are most evident in Paul's later journey to Rome by ship. At this time Paul was facing charges brought against him by some Jewish leaders, and as a Roman citizen he had invoked his right to have his case heard by the emperor. Acts 27 tells that Paul and some other prisoners were assigned to a Roman centurion, who had them board a ship bound for Italy. After sailing for some days, they experienced a terrible storm, attempted mutiny of the sailors onboard, near sinking of their ship at sea, and finally being wrecked on a reef off the Island of Malta. When we consider the difficulty of travel in his day, we can see that Paul's missionary journeys were highly strenuous and often dangerous.

The point I want to underscore here is that Paul's personal and spiritual bond with the congregations he encountered in his wide-ranging, physically, emotionally, and spiritually demanding travels as a missionary was extraordinarily strong. Many of these congregations Paul himself had founded. But even in the church at Rome, which he had not founded, there were dear friends and coworkers with whom he had close ties (Rom 16:1–15). In some sense, these congregations were his children. Paul never married and was celibate. But he had helped birth and nurture a good number of Christian congregations around the Mediterranean. One way he continued to nurture the congregations he had established was to send them letters giving instruction, critique, and encouragement.

He addressed one such letter to the Galatian Christians. The people called Galatians were a Celtic ethnic group that had migrated from Europe several centuries earlier and settled in a large region around the ancient city of Ancyra, which became the capitol of the Roman province of Galatia and today is Ankara in the central part of Turkey. The occasion for Paul's letter to them is a major change that has come about in the Galatian churches.

## Our Entry into Extended Caregiving

What appears to have occurred is that some Jewish Christians came to the Galatian churches with a different form of the Christian message than Paul preached. These Jewish Christian missionaries taught that in addition to belief in Jesus, full Christian faith involved circumcision for the men. The fact that some of the Galatian Christians adopted this view troubles Paul greatly. He states baldly, "Listen! I, Paul, am telling you that if you let yourselves be circumcised, Christ will be of no benefit to you. . . . For in Christ Jesus neither circumcision nor uncircumcision counts for anything; the only thing that counts is faith working through love" (Gal 5:2, 6).

### Christ Present with Us

We may readily agree that faith in Christ rather than our good works is the key to right relationship with God. This is a familiar message that we may have heard time and again. However, Paul also has another, much less familiar message that is profoundly relevant for caregiving. This less familiar message comes to expression in these words: "I have been crucified with Christ; and it is no longer I who live, but it is Christ who lives in me. And the life I now live in the flesh I live by faith in the Son of God, who loved me and gave himself for me" (Gal 2:19-20).

In his monumental study *The Theology of Paul the Apostle*, highly respected British New Testament scholar James D. G. Dunn says of this and similar expressions from other Pauline writings:

> Paul evidently felt himself to be caught up "in Christ" and borne along by Christ. In some sense he experienced Christ as the context of all his being and doing. We can hardly avoid some sort of locative sense in the preposition "in," at least in a number of cases. What that might mean for his Christology is a subject to which we must return. Here we focus more on the evident sense of Christ's presence as more or less a constant factor, from within which Paul consciously and subconsciously drew resource and strength for all his activities.[7]

*For Paul, this sense of Christ's presence is not primarily a doctrine, an idea, but an experience.* The difference between an idea and an experience is like the difference between *talking about* being in love and *actually being* in love. The experiential reality of actually being in love colors one's thoughts and motivation in a profound way. Similarly, for Paul "being in Christ" is an

---

7. Dunn, *The Theology of Paul the Apostle* (Grand Rapids: Eerdmans, 1998), 400.

experiential reality that colors one's thoughts, feelings, and actions. If I am in Christ, I am not alone in facing difficulty or success. Christ is *with* me.

Indeed, James Dunn strengthens this perspective when he says a complementary feature in Paul's letters is his "with Christ" motif. Paul's expression "with Christ" appears in about forty compound words such as, "For if we have been united with him in a death like his, we will certainly be united with him in a resurrection like his. We know that our old self was crucified with him" (Rom 6:5–6). Dunn says Paul's many "in Christ" and "with Christ" phrases are meant "to express the same sense of a communality of believers rooted in its dependence upon their common experience of participation in Christ."[8]

Dunn emphasizes that Paul's language of being "in Christ" and "with Christ" cannot be reduced to merely a feature of Pauline *literary style*. Rather, in these expressions the more mystical dimension of Christ's life, death, and resurrection comes to the fore. Dunn also says this language cannot be reduced simply to a description of baptism or of membership in the believing community, the church. For you and me to be "in Christ" and "with Christ" is to live moment by moment in Christ's presence. We are not alone. Christ is with us.[9]

Consider the implications of this "mystical dimension" for our caregiving today. When we are the primary caregiver not just for a few hours now and then, but throughout most or even all of the day and every day, we get tired. Really tired. And when we get really tired, we tend to become irritable, and finally explode. But if we are not alone in caregiving, the burden is shared. If we have a family member or dear friend share the burden now and then or have someone we hire to give in-home assistance a few hours a week, we know what a relief that is. But even with much valued assistance from others, the primary responsibility week in and week out is still on us. That takes its toll.

Since God is always present, there is always the potential of being open to the divine presence, of turning to that gracious presence at any time of day or night. In one interview with a recent widow, I remarked:

---

8. Dunn, *Theology of Paul*, 403.

9. "Paul's language indicates rather a quite profound sense of participation with others in a great and cosmic movement of God centered on Christ and effected through his Spirit. Here again a term like 'mysticism' is only an attempt to indicate that profundity and to signal that there are depths and resonances here which we may not be able fully to explore, but for which we need to keep our ears attuned." Dunn, *Theology of Paul*, 404.

## Our Entry into Extended Caregiving

"You said you pray a lot? Any particular practices?"

She said, "I'm a prayer whisperer. Do you know what I mean?"

Brad: "No."

She said, "Not formal and sit down and pray. But those momentary prayers. You find yourself saying, 'What am I going to do now? Here's where I need your help, Lord.' Whisper prayers. That's what I always call them. I've never been a big formal pray-er. But a prayer whisperer—throughout the day, and sometimes (soft laugh), throughout the night. I feel supported and helped along the way."

Notice that she says "I feel supported and helped along the way."

I asked another woman, who is the primary caregiver for her mother with Lewy body dementia, "What role, if any, have your personal faith and spiritual practice played in your caregiving?"

She replied:

> Well, I don't know how people do it without faith. That is definitely a lifeline for me. I know that I am not alone in this journey, nor is my mom alone in those times when she cannot connect with us. I know that God holds her. That's huge, just *huge*. My practice of daily devotions each day is to read Scripture, centering prayer, and journaling. It's a way to God's hand in time."

Notice she says, "It's a way to God's hand in time." This woman's devotional practices are her way of reaching out to God's supporting hand.

Not only is God able to be *with us* in every situation, over time God is also able to nurture in us those qualities needed to provide the most beneficial care. Paul identifies many of these qualities in his letter to the Galatians when he calls this community of Christians to exhibit the "fruit of the Spirit." In his instruction to the Galatian Christians, Paul draws a sharp contrast between "the works of the flesh" and "the fruit of the Spirit." He says:

> Now the works of the flesh are obvious: fornication, impurity, licentiousness, idolatry, sorcery, enmities, strife, jealousy, anger, quarrels, dissensions, factions, envy, drunkenness, carousing, and things like these. I am warning you, as I warned you before: those who do such things will not inherit the kingdom of God. By contrast, the fruit of the Spirit is love, joy, peace, patience, kindness, generosity, faithfulness, gentleness, and self-control. (Gal 5:19–23)

Since Paul's attention is focused on the *community* of Galatian Christians, his instruction centers on those personal attributes that break down a Christian community and those attributes that build up that community. First, Paul's list of sins here covers four categories of sin. Fornication, impurity, and licentiousness are sexual sins; idolatry and sorcery are sins of religious practice; and drunkenness and carousing are excessive use of alcohol. But Paul gives his fullest attention to those sins that specifically undermine personal relationships and community: "enmities, strife, jealousy, anger, quarrels, dissensions, factions." James Dunn underscores Paul's focus in this passage and in parts of his other letters on those sins that undermine community:

> Two features are worth noting. One is that the bulk of the vices listed are social. The effect of sin is seen at its most serious not so much in secret vices practiced in private, but in the breakdown of human relationships. The other is that so many of the vices are petty—the petty acts of envy and deceit, of jealousy and conceit, of gossip and backbiting, of greed and spite, of heartlessness and ruthlessness. But it is precisely such petty vices which undermine a community of trust and poison society.[10]

Corresponding to Paul's special concern for the Galatian *community* is his list of the fruit of the Spirit in Galatians 5:22–23: "love, joy, peace, patience, kindness, generosity, faithfulness, gentleness, and self-control." The last of these—self-control—was an ancient prescription for excessive use of alcohol. We now have a deeper understanding of alcoholism as an addiction, which an individual is commonly unable to control without special support. But the other fruit of the Spirit identified by Paul make for constructive, supportive, durable caregiving. These are personal qualities—what ethicists call *virtues*. It is to these "fruit of the Spirit" that our attention turns. The first is love.

---

10. Dunn, *Theology of Paul*, 124.

CHAPTER THREE

# Love

THE NEW TESTAMENT USES three different Greek words that are translated into English as "love." The Greek word *phileo* refers to the love between friends, as in Philadelphia, which has been traditionally rendered as "the city of brotherly love." Corresponding to love as passion is the ancient Greek notion of love as *eros*, which refers to the desire and longing to possess. This can be sexual desire as in the English derivative "erotic." But *eros* can also refer to one's strong attachment to chocolate cake or a certain kind of music. The third Greek word for love is *agape*, which is developed in the New Testament as love that seeks the beloved's well-being and is deeply faithful and generously forgiving.

In Galatians 5:22 Paul identifies the first "fruit of the Spirit" as *agape* love. Several caregivers I interviewed expressed *agape* love without using the word "love." My opening question to the still active caregivers I interviewed was: "Describe your caregiving situation as it is today." One woman, whose husband with Parkinson's is now in a nursing home, responded, "I think today it is to do what I can, when I go to visit him, to make *his* day as good as it can be." And near the end of the interview she said:

> When you've been with a person for years, and done so many things together, and depended on each other, it's pretty hard to just drop that. I think it's a privilege. It's the love that you can continue to show. People have said, "Doesn't going there twice a day get to be too much for you?" Sometimes I don't stay as long as other days, but some days I'll stay two-and-half hours if he needs me to be there. I don't feel it's a drudgery at all or anything like that at all.

> You do as much as you possibly can to make it better for them as you can. Knowing that they're sitting there *hours* by themselves.

Another spouse of a husband with Parkinson's said, "I suppose by the last five years of his life, it became more my responsibility to see that he was getting through each day the best that he could."

A daughter described her father's care for her mother who has Lewy body dementia.

> Everything he did was focused on, "What is best for _____? How can I provide the best care for her?" I get very tearful, just the loyalty and dedication. If someone would ask me, "What does love look like?" I would point to Dad. His whole life, but especially in those last years, when Mom was in the care facility and not able to give back to the relationship. She sometimes has moments of being combative. Literally emptying yourself as a servant to someone and then have them treat you poorly. That would be so hard.

*Agape* love, seeking to do "what is best for" our loved one with dementia, requires some knowledge of our loved one's medical condition. Several of the caregivers I interviewed spoke with appreciation of the helpful information on the disease provided by the national organization on Alzheimer's or Parkinson's. For instance, understanding that a person with dementia may become combative, even physically striking others, can enable one to remain calm and respond in a helpful way. So, for instance, a son began to sing a hymn when his aged mother with advanced Alzheimer's became agitated and combative. Singing hymns familiar to her and with her, one after another, calmed her.

*Agape* love also came through in the remarks of a widow who had a long, rather contentious marriage with her husband who developed dementia with Lewy bodies and was in a nursing home for the final year-and-a-half of his life.

> Brad: "When we talked before, you said that when [he] was in the nursing home, you went to visit him every day for one hour. A lot of people who have had a difficult relationship with a person would just ignore that person, not visit them. You two had a difficult relationship, but you went to visit him every day for an hour. Why was that? Why did you do that?"
>
> Widow: "I just wanted to go. Even though he wasn't nice to me . . . He wasn't even nice to me *there* [at the nursing home]."

Brad: "Well, I've wondered about that, why you visited him every day."

Widow: "I guess that's who I am: forgiving people. I even did *want* to go."

*Agape* love also animates another person's care for his mother, who has late-stage Alzheimer's, and for his father, who has mid-stage Parkinson's disease. He visits them every day. When he described his involvement with them, I said, "That's pretty extensive involvement then, isn't it?" He replied,

> I was talking about this with [my wife] a couple weeks ago. There was someone . . . who said, "It must be a great burden." But I find it kind of relieving, because before, when they lived [at another place] . . . I had to drive two hours going and two hours returning, once a week. And every time I left there, I felt anxious about not seeing them for a week. I always remind myself what a mercy it is that I can see them every day.

*Agape* love also pervades the reflections of this man whose wife had been diagnosed recently with "unspecified dementia type without behavioral disturbance." When I asked whether he thought of caring for her as a privilege or a duty, he replied,

> I was a caregiver, I was a physician. My feeling has been simply this—that I've been given the most important patient of my life, to take care of her. I feel that it's partly a duty—I made a vow—but that really doesn't come into it. This person is an extension of me. It's my privilege to do all that I can, to make what life there is left, the best it can possibly be under the circumstances.
>
> She is in continual grief, and I can tell it. She had to leave choir; she couldn't remember things. She watches the choir, and I know she wants to be there. She can't play bridge, and she *knows* she can't play bridge. She feels some of her friends have sort of abandoned her. I don't think they have, but she feels . . . she feels she's less of a person than she was.
>
> It's a privilege, a challenge to me. I feel I'm being monitored, and I don't feel bad about being monitored. Are you doing the most you can to make this most important patient in your life as comfortable as possible? Yes, we have little flare-ups. She has the cognition and understanding to know that. This is the job that I really and truly want to do.
>
> My life was known from the beginning; not known to me, but it was known. Every one of us that's here on earth has hit the

biological jackpot. The chances of our being here, the chances of that particular little sperm getting to her egg. There were thousands of other sperm and they would be other people. Each of us has hit the jackpot of life. The gift of life is so precious. I thank the Lord for my life. This is a job that I *care* to do. It's a job that I *want* to do. Sure, it's a job, but it's a job I want to do. There may be times that I feel it's a duty, but it's a duty that I want to do. Sure, at times it's frustrating. Damn it. It's not what you're given, but what you make of what you're given. If I outlive her, I'm going to say, "Thank God for that." Because it made our last years better, closer together. And I wouldn't have to say, "I should have spent more of our life together."

In fact, it was true of everyone I interviewed that their caregiving was animated by *agape* love. Those who were non-religious also demonstrated self-giving love for their family member. One set of a non-religious son and daughter of their widowed mother both made major changes in their own lives, in order to care for their mother and keep her, as she wished, in her own home. The son gave up his job and home, in order to move to his mother's city, find a new job, and take care of her. When the son's health seriously declined, the daughter moved halfway across the country to assume caregiving for him and their mother. They both exhibited *agape* love.

Indeed, those for whom these self-giving people provide care are the fortunate ones among those who need care. One caregiver, who was visiting her husband daily in a care facility, commented:

> Some people don't have anyone visit. And they have family, but they don't come. I know they have family here, but they don't come. Then you see them coming. Lo and behold, that's when they're dying. They don't come to see them when they're still living and how excited they are when they see you.
>
> As I've been going back and forth, I've been able to give a little bit of cheer to some of these people. I know there's a gentleman who was in assisted living. I know he has children here, but you don't see anyone visiting very often. And they're all right around here. But they don't come. Every time I'd come in that entrance to assisted living and then go into the nursing home area. And often he was sitting there. I think he knew I was coming and was sitting there, so he could have somebody to talk with. He was looking forward to it. That's too bad. That gentleman probably had me visit with him for a few minutes, and that may have been the only company he had all day.

# Love

It is not accidental that the first fruit of the Spirit that Paul mentions in Galatians 5:22 is *agape* love, for in his understanding, love is foundational for living well. In his first letter to the Christian congregation in Corinth Paul expresses his grand praise of *agape* love:

> If I speak in the tongues of mortals and of angels, but do not have love, I am a noisy gong or a clanging cymbal. And if I have prophetic powers, and understand all mysteries and all knowledge, and if I have all faith, so as to remove mountains, but do not have love, I am nothing. If I give away all my possessions, and if I hand over my body so that I may boast, but do not have love, I gain nothing.
>
> Love is patient; love is kind; love is not envious or boastful or arrogant or rude. It does not insist on its own way; it is not irritable or resentful; it does not rejoice in wrongdoing, but rejoices in the truth. It bears all things, believes all things, hopes all things, endures all things.
>
> Love never ends. But as for prophecies, they will come to an end; as for tongues, they will cease; as for knowledge, it will come to an end. (1 Cor 13:1–8)

The centrality of *agape* love in the Christian life is fundamental for Paul. The religious life of many first-century Christians included ecstatic experiences such as speaking in tongues and prophecies, yet he implies that it is possible to use such rapturous experiences in a self-serving manner. Even becoming a martyr for the faith could be done for self-aggrandizement. True love is kind, it benefits others. New Testament scholar James Dunn says of this passage in 1 Corinthians:

> It is hard to doubt that Paul in thus describing love had in mind the love of God in Christ, and Jesus' own summary of the law in the command to love the neighbor. A similar inference is appropriate in his naming love as the primary or all-embracing fruit of the Spirit (Gal. 5:22-23). It is just this love which identifies and defines the Spirit as the Spirit of Christ, the Spirit of the self-giving and crucified Christ.[1]

Because such love is foundational for good caregiving, we have to be prudent in nurturing a loving spirit. Some very practical, down-to-earth provisions make it more likely that we caregivers can act out of love. The most basic provision is to get adequate rest. We are physical beings whose

---

1. Dunn, *Theology of Paul*, 596.

bodily condition powerfully influences how we behave. Fatigue saps our spirit of love. Getting adequate rest often requires planning. Sometimes this planning involves hired help. Other times, if circumstances permit, family members may assist.

In my situation, I turned first to our three children for rest and temporary relief from caregiving Marion. In the following email exchanges, first I appealed to them for help with Marion's care and later I sought their advice about my own mental condition.

*Brad to Julie, Carter, Kim, September 17, 2018*

I'm going to need your help in caregiving Mom over the coming year. It is critical for me that I get sufficient rest. My experience has been that after three months, I become more tired, and the accompanying increased irregularity in my sleep pattern adds greatly to the fatigue. This makes it vital that periodically I get away for a retreat and deep rest. Julie is scheduled to come again this Friday (September 21–23) while I go away on retreat. She also did this late last spring.

Looking ahead, I'm hoping that Carter may be able to come again for two days just prior to Christmas, as you did last year. Looking further ahead, I hope that Kim may be able to come for a forty-eight-hour period sometime, say, in March. I realize, Kim, that you and Bryce are coming here for Thanksgiving, and a while ago you and Bryce were here for Christmas. I don't want to go away on a retreat when Bryce is here, so I'm hoping that you can work out coming alone sometime in March.

Love,

Dad

*Brad to Julie, Carter, Kim, October 29, 2018*

Julie, Carter, Kim,

Things are going quite well for Mom and me. The most significant factor that I want to call to your attention is that I'm aware that I am not as mentally sharp as I once was. The large book that I have open now before me is titled *Mayo Clinic on Alzheimer's Disease*, and while it focuses on Alzheimer's, it also treats a good number of other conditions that cause dementia: Parkinson's, Dementia with Lewy Bodies, and various vascular disorders such as a series of small strokes (Grandma Hanson had this), and distinguishes all these diseases from "typical aging." The book says that as we age our brain actually shrinks in size, and our mind is not as nimble as it once was. Some aspects of forgetfulness that come with typical aging are: difficulty recalling details (e.g., title of a book, a friend's birthday), being absent minded (can't find something, forget an appointment), memory blocks (can't come up with the words to express what you want to say), and making sense of new or unfamiliar information may be more difficult.

Of course, like nearly everybody else my age, often I can't come up with the name of a person, film, or book that I'm talking about. We old duffers (Mary Lou and Martin Mohr, Harlan Nelson, Will Bunge, Dennis Barnaal, etc.) over morning coffee at Luther often commiserate and chuckle together about this.

The recent events that have especially brought this to my attention include: having a check returned from a charity, because I had not signed it; missing the proper exit off I-694 going to Jerry's funeral (Trudi's husband) a few weeks ago.

As I say, I don't think this is anything to worry about. It's just "typical aging," and you will likely experience some of this soon, if not already. But it does mean that it would be helpful for you to be observant, so that I don't screw up in a major way.

Love,

Dad

*Carter to Brad, October 30, 2018*

Hi Dad,

I would agree that the symptoms you describe are just "typical aging" and nothing more serious. Michelle and I are already experiencing some of that too. It's harder for us to come up with names of people than it used to be, stuff like that. It's mostly just mildly frustrating rather than being truly worrisome.

Love to you and Mom,

Carter

# Finding Grace in Caregiving

*Julie to Brad, November 2, 2018*

>Hi Dad,
>
>Sorry for not responding earlier. I've been on vacation this week and have been avoiding email.
>
>We have also noticed things with your memory over the last couple of years, such as forgetting to bring things when you visit, forgetting details (as you mentioned), sometimes asking about something we talked about a little while ago. I also find my memory is not as sharp as it once was. Have you ever considered getting checked out just to make sure it's not something more than typical aging?
>
>We're looking forward to seeing you and Mom (and everyone else) for Thanksgiving. I'm still planning on bringing a couple of pies. Please let me know if there's anything else we can bring.
>
>Love,
>
>Julie

Having strong support every few months from our three adult children is a huge benefit for Marion and me. If I had to do sustained caregiving of Marion all alone, I would collapse. Then both of us would be in need of care.

In addition to help from our children, starting in May 2019 I arranged to have a professional care worker come to our home for just two or three hours a week to do some cleaning. Although early on Marion bristled at this other woman's alien presence in our home, after several weeks she became more comfortable with Sharon, a CNA, who with my encouragement engaged Marion's participation in various tasks.

I think we caregivers not only need support from others, at times we also need to be self-critical. Some of our behavior, that we may think is loving, may actually arise out of our own personal need. A case in point is this man, who tells about his care for his wife with advanced cancer.

> I was going with her to Mayo frequently for radiation. At home she spent most of the days in bed. Her weight was going down. Every time she weighed in, her weight had gone down. That was devastating to me. I knew how important good nutrition is for maintaining weight. I provided whatever she wanted to eat. But often she asked just for macaroni and cheese, which isn't great in

nutrition. One time I prepared that, and afterward I saw that she hadn't eaten much. I felt profound grief.

I did my typical thing. I thought, "I have to bring it up to her."

She said, "Well, I just can't eat more."

But as time went on, I'd bring it up again, like a broken record, as gentle and loving as I could be, concerned. Then she'd express annoyance with me. She suffered for years with esophageal reflux. She said, "I don't want to have any more supper." That was unacceptable to me.

Then I had a sudden awareness. This matter is not about food. It's about watching your wife die. You're helpless. Of course, there was denial too. So the truth is that you're losing her. *That changed everything.* It was really *my* problem. For me that was a breakthrough. That released me from that issue, so I could be more caringly present to her. That was one of the major emotional crises I went through.

It is not accidental that in describing the fruit of the Spirit Paul begins with *agape* love, because *agape*'s concern for the well-being of others is fundamental for all gifts of the Spirit. So having laid the foundation in *agape* love for the Galatian Christian community, Paul goes on to his next fruit of the Spirit—joy.

CHAPTER FOUR

# Joy

IT IS NOT SURPRISING that Paul next calls the attention of the Galatian Christians to joy, for the emphasis of the "Judaizers" on strict observance of the law could squeeze joy out of religious life. But what does joy have to do with us who do caregiving, particularly caregiving someone with memory loss? When we are in a long-term caregiving situation, how are the caregiver and recipient of care to have joy? Especially when we are in an end-of-life caregiving situation that may last several years, what is there to be joyful about? The reality of long-term caregiving of a loved one is that sadness and grief are frequent and persistent companions.

One of the little daily rituals that Marion and I share when we are home is a short devotion a few minutes before we eat our evening meal. We use a book that gives a Scripture text for the day, a brief commentary on that biblical text, a hymn from the Lutheran Book of Worship, and a short concluding prayer. I read aloud the Scripture text and brief commentary on it. Then Marion reads aloud the words of the suggested hymn text. Frequently now when Marion reads the hymn text, she stumbles over some words and phrases. When this happens, I feel a tug at my heart, and sometimes I fight to hold back tears. It grieves me to hear this woman, who once was so intelligent, falter in this elemental way.

Indeed, the reason I first became aware of her very existence was seeing her name, a student from my hometown, listed among the new members of the prestigious academic honor society Phi Beta Kappa at my college alma mater. I immediately consulted a college yearbook from a recent graduate and I saw that she was pretty. Smart and pretty—I was going to check her out. Several weeks later I visited my parents in my hometown, and I called

Marion for a date. She agreed. We went on a double date with some of my friends, and the very next evening she and I had a picnic by ourselves. Going into her house after that second date, she said to her mother, "That is the man I am going to marry." I was a bit slower. It took me about five weeks to know that she was the one for me.

My appreciation of Marion's intelligence and beauty has been renewed often through the years. One especially memorable instance occurred sometime during the early 1990s when Marion was leading an Alzheimer's support group for Area Agency on Aging. I was probably on spring break from classes at Luther College when she invited me to go with her to the Alzheimer's support group in a neighboring county. After setting up tables and chairs in a square, Marion greeted people as they arrived and then stood up to begin the session. Sitting down and looking up at her from the side, I saw her from a fresh perspective. She replied to people's comments and questions with clear, thoughtful answers. And man, was she beautiful! It reminded me of how powerfully she had touched me when we first met. However, now more than four decades later, to hear this very bright woman struggle during our daily devotions to read aloud a hymn text line broke my heart.

An especially painful moment came on an early May 2018 evening after supper, when Marion and I sat out on our deck. I began to tell her about an email I had sent to three old friends reporting on some ideas about contemporary journalism recently expressed in a Luther College public lecture by Ted Koppel, the former ABC news anchor. Koppel had bemoaned the decline of journalism grounded in the hard work of gathering *facts*, which is labor intensive and expensive. What has largely replaced it in the United States, according to Koppel, is the far less costly version of "news" consisting of panelists expressing their *opinions*. Marion had been with me at the Koppel lecture. So, assuming some shared familiarity with Koppel's ideas, I began to tell Marion about the content of my email to these old friends. She never said a word of comment or question. In fact, she barely made a sound. After a few minutes my heart sank; it dawned on me that she was no longer able to discuss such an issue. My sense of loss was deep. Our ability to discuss issues in contemporary culture and religion has been a staple of our life together. To be sure, our ability to have such conversations had been declining gradually for several years, but on this evening, her almost total lack of response to my comments produced a deep sadness in me. And I realized that this was not the end of her decline. I knew that more heart break lay ahead. Dementia brings an enormous weight of sadness. How then can Marion find joy in this situation? How can I as her caregiver find joy? Although dementia gradually squeezes the joy out of life, it is vital for all concerned that we caregivers nurture as much joy as possible.

We can be guided by Saint Paul, who endured great suffering in his own life, and was sensitive to the hardship and suffering of others, yet often spoke of joy. *What were his grounds for joy?* Among the New Testament letters that are commonly attributed to Paul, the letter that emphasizes joy most strongly is his letter to the Philippians. Paul composed this letter to the church in Philippi while he was in prison.[1] In spite of his own very difficult circumstances, Paul uses the noun "joy" and the verb "rejoice" a total of sixteen times in this letter. It is helpful to note that his *grounds* for joy in this epistle are varied, just as the grounds for our joy vary.

At least five sources of joy may be distinguished.

*First, a valued, positive personal relationship is a common source of joy. Loving relationships within the family and good friendships are frequent occasions for joy.* Joy may be found in sharing communication and activities that are up-building for the valued relationship, such as a good heart-to-heart talk or just washing dishes in a companionate way after a meal or party. Seeing a dear family member or friend in person is often an occasion for joy, and the joy is heightened when reunion comes after a lengthy separation. Thus, Paul sends Epaphroditus back to his Philippian community, "in order that you may rejoice at seeing him again, and that I may be less anxious. Welcome him then in the Lord with all joy." Akin to this is the joy of uplifting communication with distant friends or loved ones, as Paul says, "I hope in the Lord Jesus to send Timothy to you soon, so that I may be cheered by news of you" (Phil 2:19).

Although Marion's Alzheimer's is now in the second of three stages and moving toward that final stage, she still finds several sources of joy in life, albeit with gradually diminishing scope. Her chief source of joy is found in close personal relationships. At the center of this is the relationship Marion and I have with one another. After fifty-six years of marriage, I still love Marion, and she still loves me. Although I normally rise earlier than Marion, most weekdays she is up before I leave home for my college

---

1. Although the letter makes clear that Paul is in prison when writing, it is not evident which city he is in. Scholars have argued for Rome, Ephesus, Corinth, or Caesarea, but we cannot be sure of the location.

office, and we always embrace, kiss, and bask in one another's smile before I leave. Indeed, we kiss and hug many times a day, and still find pleasure in making love.

At times Marion's desire to be close to me finds touching expression. For instance, on Friday morning, June 8, 2018 as I was just about to leave home for my college office, she came to me, gave me a hug, and said, "I just want to be near you." The following Tuesday morning soon after I'd dressed, had breakfast, and was brushing my teeth, she got out of bed to go to the bathroom. She gave me a hug and said, "Can you come back to bed?" I answered, "I'm leaving now for my office." She said, "I just want to be near you." I lay down with her for a while.

Although Marion in the second stage of Alzheimer's is unable to consistently identify our family members by name or family relationship (e.g., in the summer of 2017 she called our daughter her cousin), she still has a strong emotional connection with each of them. So she treasures a visit, phone call, or Facetime conversation with them. Marion also has a special emotional tie with her long-time local friend, Agnes, who also has significant memory loss. On occasion when Ag left after church without speaking with her, Marion wondered whether Ag was angry with her. Having Ag over for tea in an afternoon brings smiles to Marion's face. However, on one occasion, although Ag had accepted Marion's invitation to come for afternoon tea, Ag never showed; she had simply forgotten. In such an emotionally unreliable world for Marion, I feel extra strong motivation to be reliably kind with her.

This deep human need for personal connection spotlights what I believe is the most fundamental ministry of caregiving—expressing regard, interest, attention, affection, love, thereby helping the person feel that he or she matters to us. Kind words of affection and appropriate touch especially count. For family members, loving touch is powerful. Kissing and embracing Marion often is fundamental to my caregiving.

As several people I interviewed noted, some nursing home residents are virtually abandoned by their family members until the resident is dying. Especially in such cases, kind attention and amicable words from careworkers and family and friends of other residents are highly valued. Our kind presence can bring joy to a person in need of personal connection. Being kindly present—this is the very heart of the ministry of caregiving for stranger, acquaintance, friend, and loved one.

*A second source of joy is participation in a valued interest, activity, or commitment.* Friends share some common interests. A happy couple enjoys doing certain activities together. Parents who love music like to see their kids love music; parents who love golf are glad when their son or daughter enjoys golf also. In Saint Paul's case, the gospel is the highest good. So, immediately after his customary opening salutation, Paul writes, "I thank my God every time I remember you, constantly praying with joy in every one of my prayers for all of you, because of your sharing in the gospel from the first day until now" (Phil 1:3–4). Since Paul regards the gospel as the most precious good, the fact that the Philippian community shares in the gospel is an occasion for Paul's joy.

When I asked the wife of a man with significant memory impairment to describe the major changes in their caregiving situation over time, she replied:

> Ah, I guess I would say this has been at least a twelve-year process. I'll call it a "process." I think we've had to adjust . . . to *continuing narrowing* to what we can do. . . . We're in a narrowed status. There are lots of things that we can't do, and we don't do. We recognize that, and we try to start every day positively. It doesn't always work, but usually it does . . .
>
> He made decisions not to go hunting anymore. He'd gone hunting every year since college, with his sons and sons-in-law. They're all hunters. He said there were too many people that he didn't know hunting with the group. He was just not happy with it. He hasn't gone fishing in summer with ____. So an end to the hunting; an end to the fishing. He just wants to be with me.

When I asked, "What have been the major challenges that you experience in caregiving?" she answered, "I think traveling is a challenge more and more. We still insist on going, going west or east, but it's a challenge. It's disorienting and frightening. I'm getting anxious myself about traveling east and south. . . . We get frightened. So those things are challenging."

Narrowing and diminishment also describe the experience that Marion and I have had over the last ten years. As the one personally experiencing gradual cognitive decline, Marion has had to pare back, and in some cases totally give up, social connections, activities, and interests that she had previously enjoyed. For more than forty years we had enjoyed being part of a four-couple group that met monthly for an evening of conversation, a game, food, and drink, but we dropped out in 2017, because it was too hard for Marion to participate well in the evening game.

## JOY

Marion has also experienced diminishment in other activities. She enjoyed knitting for many years. However, since she has lost the ability to knit something as complicated as a prayer shawl, Marion only knits some on her own during the evening and no longer meets with our congregation's monthly prayer shawl group that she herself initiated in the early 2000s. Marion also frequently used to play solitaire while watching television with me in the evenings, but now she has entirely given that up. She still meets monthly with our congregation's women's contemplative prayer circle that she started about twenty years ago, although she no longer takes a leadership role. At this point Marion and I are also able to experience quiet joy in sharing a commitment to the Christian faith, our church, and some social bonds. Our daily suppertime brief devotion together and regular worship with our congregation are still staples of our shared life.

A social group in which Marion has found joy is the Menders. Since the late 1960s, except when she was working full time, Marion has been a regular participant in the local weekly coffee group called the Menders. They called themselves Menders because in the group's early days they were young mothers who sometimes actually mended rips and holes in family clothing. Now this group of ten to twelve old women ordinarily meets on Thursday afternoons from two to four o'clock. In an informal way, they rotate responsibility by having individuals volunteer to host or they go to a restaurant. On Thursday August 17, 2018, Marion hosted the group. Actually, the week before, she jumped the gun; thinking she was going to host that week, she had baked a lemon cake. (I was glad to see that she was still able to make this ready-mix cake, because on occasion the end product of her baking had been inedible.) When she learned that someone else had already volunteered to host, Marion said she would host the following week. So we put her frosted cake in the freezer. The following Tuesday, thinking that the Menders were coming the next day, she took the cake out of the freezer and was preparing to put pieces on plates. I told her that she was two days early, but the cake would still be fresh enough. At Thursday noon, Menders day, she did not recall how to load our large coffee maker, so together we put coffee and water in it. She already had pieces of cake on individual small plates. A half hour prior to the two o'clock start, I started the coffee maker and left for my college library office. When I returned at 4:00 all but one of the women had gone, and Marion and her last guest were bringing plates and cups to the kitchen for washing. Marion was pleased with how things had gone. Obviously hosting the Menders was important to her, and she was glad that she had done it.

Yet her memory loss made it impossible for her to hold onto her joy in hosting this group. This became evident later that same day. After supper Marion and I watched television for two hours in our family room downstairs. As we turned off the TV, I hugged her and said, "I'll bet you're really tired after hosting Menders today."

Marion: "I did?"

Me: "Yes."

Marion: "When?"

Me: "Today."

Marion: "I don't remember."

Diminishment has also struck our ability to travel, mostly because Marion's ability to drive safely has become too uncertain. Up through 2016 her driving was fine. On long trips we would alternate driving. We alternated for visits to our son, Carter, and his family in Valparaiso, Indiana, a six-hour drive. We alternated also on longer trips, driving annually for fifteen years from our home in northern Iowa to Houston, Texas. In late summer 2016, we alternated driving our granddaughter Sophie to start her freshman year at Mount Holyoke College in western Massachusetts. Around home, Marion continued to drive our second car around our town of 8000 people. But midway through 2017, I decided it was too risky for her to continue driving, and she put up only minor, very short-term resistance. My decision was not triggered by her having an accident or getting lost. It was her increased hesitancy in understanding traffic signs and traffic flow that gave me pause. While we managed well enough in 2018 to fly to Los Angeles and Seattle, it appeared too difficult in 2019. So, diminishment in travel, as well as a reduction in time together with distant family and friends, has occurred.

*A third widely shared source of joy is accomplishment of some intended goal that we value.* We are happy when a beloved child not only participates in a mutually valued activity, but participates at a high level. Parents who appreciate music are glad when their child performs well in a school musical production. Parents who love golf will be especially glad when their son or daughter becomes a varsity player on their high school team. If we value academic achievement, we're glad when we or a loved one graduates with distinction from an academic program. So in some cases in his letter to the Philippians, Paul's joy is occasioned, at least in part, by the vitality of the Philippian Christian community. He thanks them, for "in the early days of the gospel, when I left Macedonia, no church shared with me in the matter of giving and receiving, except you alone. For even when I was in Thessalonica, you sent me help for my needs more than once" (4:15–16). The goal that Marion and I have shared most fully has been rearing our children. A deep satisfaction that Marion and I feel is with our three children, who are now middle-aged. They have all graduated from college and built a successful career, each in a different line of work. Yet Marion's joy in our children's accomplishments is fitful and muted, because she needs to be reminded of what they have done.

*A fourth and especially poignant occasion for joy is escape from a threat such as major injury, serious disease, or war.* In his letter to the Philippian Christians, Paul calls attention to the joy they will have at seeing Epaphroditus on his return home, for he "was indeed so ill that he nearly died" (Phil 2:27). For those of us doing end of life caregiving or caregiving a person with an incurable condition, there may be joy for getting through a difficult episode, but there is no escape from the underlying condition. In this respect, we can only find a sober joy in the hope for life beyond death.

*A fifth source of joy, not mentioned by Paul in his letter to the Philippian congregation, is found in basic physical pleasures such as a good meal, a favorite drink, a beautiful view, pleasing physical activity, kissing your beloved.*

Marion and I find joy in the physical circumstances of our life. We live in a beautiful, generally safe college town with many interesting cultural events. We live in our own home that we had built on a street called Ridge Road, that winds its way along a hilltop ridge that on both sides falls away into woods. Midway through almost every afternoon when we enjoy a cup of tea together, we gaze into the wooded area behind our house. Of course, the view changes with each of the four seasons, but we always find beauty to be appreciated. In fact, from time to time she comments on what a beautiful view we have. After tea, we either take a two-mile walk, usually in our neighborhood, or engage in some outside work.

While some people engage in physical activity such as taking a walk or going to a gym only because they feel they *ought*, Marion and I are fortunate in that we genuinely enjoy walking and much of the other physical activity we regularly do. Indeed, it is not accidental that certain forms of physical activity are called *work*, while other forms are called *recreation—re-creation*. Granted, I do not find as much enjoyment and recreation in a two-mile walk as I used to find in playing tennis. For me tennis was really fun. I thoroughly enjoyed it. I know that some people find joy mostly in winning at a game like tennis, but winning did not matter much to me. I was more pleased with losing a well-played match than winning a poorly played one. To be sure, a neighborhood walk for me is not fun like tennis, but it is usually pleasant. A good walk has re-creative power for me.

I may be crazy, but ordinarily I look forward to mowing the lawn or blowing snow off our driveway and sidewalk. And it's not just the bottle of beer or pop afterward that I look forward to. The mowing or blowing snow, even shoveling snow, is satisfying to me. Admittedly, I cannot say that I *enjoy* the inside task of cleaning our bathroom. For me these various tasks are necessary work. But they yield the bonus of giving me physical exercise that I need and want.

Underlying these specific sources of enjoyment, Marion and I are fortunate to have basic life circumstances that, given our ages, are quite good. Our income from Social Security, pensions, and retirement investments makes for a life free from financial worry. Medicare and our health insurance give us access to high quality medical care locally and world-class care at the Rochester Mayo Clinic, an eighty-minute drive away. We are very lucky to have been born when and where we were and to caring parents who encouraged education. Many people, indeed, most people in the world and the United States are not nearly so lucky. To be sure, we have both worked hard. But millions of people in the United States, as well as billions of people on earth, work hard, yet struggle to get by.

What impresses me most about Marion is that she does not grumble or lash out at God for losing her memory. Indeed, she manifests an amazing level of joy. This is helped, no doubt, by her early recognition and acceptance that Alzheimer's disease is gradually destroying her mind. From the start, she has been very clear-eyed about it. A woman in her Menders coffee group told me, "I remember when she came to Menders, we were at Aggie's, and you know, she said matter of factly, 'I have Alzheimer's.' She faces things straight on. It takes a lot of strength to do that." Sometime in 2017 was the final time I asked Marion how *she felt* about having Alzheimer's. She said very little. Most likely answering that question required a level of cognitive ability that was then beyond her. In any event, she does not mope or lash out at me or anyone else. She is cheerful and very appreciative of me. She often says that she loves me. And daily she also tells me, "You know, I sorta, kinda like you." The "sorta, kinda like" does not signal lukewarm regard. It is her particular way of expressing deep appreciation and love for me.

Experiencing joy is beneficial not only for recipients of caregiving, but also for those of us who do caregiving. Joy is especially vital, because caregiving a loved one with dementia brings with it profound sorrow. In my case, I am losing the person whom I love most in this world, who is also my best friend. I realize that I am fortunate that this loss is occurring late in our life together, rather than in an early or middle stage, as happens to some. I must admit, also, that I am lucky that my loss of Marion is occurring gradually, rather than quickly, as is the case for those who lose a loved one to accident or heart attack. Nonetheless, my experience of loss and its accompanying sadness are real and powerful.

Sadness over this gradual losing of Marion erupts sometimes without warning. One mid-August evening in 2018 Marion and I were watching a public television musical program featuring Andrea Bocelli, the blind Italian singer sometimes described as a crossover tenor, because his singing appeals to both operatic and popular audiences. Toward the end of the program Bocelli and a soprano sang a number entitled "Time to Say Goodbye," partly in Italian and partly in English. Although I could only understand the English lyrics, the song brought tears to my eyes, for it reminded me that Marion and I are in an extended time of saying goodbye. The words of a woman whose husband had died of Parkinson's after more than twenty years with the disease came back to me, "It's a very long goodbye." The reality is that Marion is gradually slipping away from me. Since I did not want Marion to see my reaction to the song, I hid my tears from her.

Our sense of loss of a personal relationship depends on the depth of our emotional investment in that relationship. We have a great variety of interactions with other people. Indeed, day to day we may see a considerable number of people. If we're in an urban setting, most of those we see may be complete *strangers* to us; we have no personal connection with them. But we encounter some people who are *acquaintances*; we know who they are and on occasion may speak with them, but we do not regularly interact with them. In addition, we may work or cooperate in a project with persons who are *associates*, but are not friends. *A friend is someone with whom we have a mutual liking*, and so we willingly choose to spend time with one another.

Yet we do not like all our friends equally. *I find it useful to distinguish among four levels of friendship: (ordinary) friend, good friend, close friend, and best friend.* Ordinary friends are those with whom we sometimes converse and do things, but we do not have a special emotional connection with them. A good friend is someone we especially value, a person with whom we share some common interests and with whom we make an effort to spend quality time. A close friend is someone with whom we share much of our inner life, our personal hopes and worries. Our best friend is the person with whom we have the deepest emotional bond.

Psychologist Beverly Fehr says that friendship serves three of our important needs—stimulation in shared activities and conversation, help and support, and love and esteem.[2]

1. The first of these aspects of friendship—stimulation in shared activities and conversation—is being steadily diminished for Marion and me. Over our years as married best friends Marion and I have shared most fully with one another in setting common goals, rearing our children, supporting our grandchildren, and managing everyday life together. We have also enjoyed discussing religious practices, theological ideas, political ideas, cultural events such as plays, movies, lectures, and current events. Currently, the daily activities we are still able to share are a trip to the supermarket, usually having lunch together, most often taking a daily walk together late in the afternoon, having dinner together, watching television in the evening, and snuggling and kissing throughout the day. We are able yet to make an occasional trip together to family members, but long trips will likely end soon. We still are able to share these activities, but a former staple of our shared life—discussion of issues and current events—has disappeared. So, one significant dimension of our long friendship has ended. What we most commonly discuss now is a shopping list for daily groceries, and even that discussion is very one sided.

2. The second dimension of friendship—help and support—has become much more one-sided than before. Until the last few years, Marion and I had always cared for and supported one another; it was entirely mutual. Gradually the balance has shifted, so that now my care and support for her has to be far more vigilant and sustained. No longer can I take off on my own for a day or two without making sure that

---

2. Fehr, *Friendship Processes* (Thousand Oaks, CA: Sage, 1996), 5.

someone else is watching over her. On her part, Marion has become much more dependent upon me for emotional support. The awareness hits me from time to time that, while God is Marion's eternal anchor, I am now her temporal anchor, her primary temporal source of stability, safety, and affirmation. The presence of her Bible and her personal wooden hand-held cross next to the easy chair in our study testify to her abiding faith in God. I know that she finds strength and stability in God, who is infinite and eternal. But her chief anchor in the ever-shifting flux of this finite, temporal world is me. Being that temporal anchor is the greatest responsibility of my life.

3. The third dimension of our friendship—love and esteem—has grown greatly. On her side, it seems to me that her love and appreciation for me has become deeper and stronger. Frequently during the day she hugs and kisses me and expresses her ironic declaration, "You know, I sorta, kinda like you." On my side, my love and esteem for her have taken on new depth. I have been and am still amazed at her open-eyed courage in facing Alzheimer's. Whereas most people afflicted with the disease begin with only a superficial understanding of it and often try to explain away their mental lapses, Marion knew from the beginning what Alzheimer's would do to her. Her earlier direct involvement with numerous persons with Alzheimer's through her work with the Area Agency on Aging showed her how the disease ravages its victims. Marion has never tried to sugarcoat her condition. She has faced it straight on, and for that I admire her tremendously.

While I am gradually losing my best friend, Marion, like many other elderly caregivers, I have fewer close friends with whom to share my caregiving burden. While any friend will express sympathy for one's difficulty, I have found that it is an unusual friend who is able to continue looking me in the eye while I express concern about Marion's dementia. Most people seem uncomfortable with the topic. This was not true of Paul. The two of us met for lunch with some regularity. While we talked about current events, we focused most on our family and our health. It was comforting for me to shared my latest caregiving experiences and concerns with him. It was comforting for me to feel that someone in addition to my kids shared my caregiving burden. One day, though, Paul told me that he had been diagnosed with colon cancer, which could not be surgically removed, only slowed down by chemotherapy. The chemo treatments were very unpleasant, but he carried on, and we continued to meet for lunch each week. By the summer of 2017, though, he was mostly confined to his condo, so I visited him there once or twice a week. Then in late October I received a phone call from his daughter saying that Paul was dying and the end was near. I immediately drove over to see him. He was unable to talk except to mumble over and over, "Goodbye, goodbye, goodbye." Since Paul's death, my caregiving burden has felt somewhat heavier.

Of course, the internet makes it possible to communicate with friends who live far away. The recent Facebook notice of my birthday elicited several notes from friends that I had not seen for a while. Simple posts from two friends with whom I had cooperated in starting and leading the two-year Grace Institute Spiritual Formation Program led to several more substantive exchanges about our current situations and hopes for the future.

Mostly through email or Facebook I stay in touch now and then with longtime friends that I'll refer to simply as C, H, and G, but nothing quite replaces being together in the same space. So, it was especially good when C and I were together for almost all of our sixtieth college reunion in June, 2017. In July, 2018, H and his wife joined Marion and me for lunch when we visited our son in Los Angeles, and when G makes his annual visit to Decorah, our weekly lunchtime conversations are especially thoughtful and emotionally rich. But any such relationship in which geographically distant friends communicate only now and then cannot have the richness of a relationship in which there is frequent in-depth face-to-face communication.

Although it is common for all elderly women and men to lose the treasured companionship of loved ones and good friends, this ever greater diminishment of social and emotional support places an especially hard burden on those of us who are also going through the gradual loss of the loved for whom we are caregiving. Extended caregiving is so taxing that we caregivers need all the support and encouragement we can get from family and friends.

Of course, Marion and I are not the only members of our family to experience the loss of her memory; so do our daughter and two sons. Since I am with her nearly every day, I have adjusted in some measure to Marion's cognitive condition in the second stage of Alzheimer's disease. Often having to repeat my verbal comments, write down daily scheduled events, and hunt for misplaced utensils in the kitchen do not feel exceptional and usually do not upset me. Since our children and grandchildren are with her only now and then, and most often when I am also present to make connections, their awareness of her decline may be less acute. But they experience disappointment and grief in some interactions with Marion, especially when I am absent. Our daughter Julie felt especially sad when visiting Marion in 2017 and Marion called Julie her cousin.

While escape from serious disease, accident, financial loss, war, or natural disaster is a source of joy for many people, there is currently no happy escape from Alzheimer's disease. Dealing with the sadness from Marion's unrelenting decline is a challenge for me and for our three children.

Facing such loss, it is well to remember a different kind of joy. The apostle Paul points us to joy that is grounded not in happy circumstances, relief from a threat, or human achievement, but entirely in God's grace. Such joy has a defiant quality about it. It can be joy *in spite of* pain, loss, and heartache. The defiance of this joy is based on God's gracious promise. The book of Acts gives striking expression to this defiant joy when it tells of the response of "Peter and the apostles" to the orders of the high priest and elders not to proclaim the resurrection of Jesus. When Peter and the apostles continue to proclaim Jesus' resurrection in spite of this dire warning, they are again brought before the high priest and elders, flogged, and ordered again not to proclaim Jesus as Messiah. Then we're told, "As they left the council, they rejoiced that they were considered worthy to suffer dishonor for the sake of the name" (Acts 5:41). Imagine, they felt joy at being *flogged* for declaring their faith in Jesus as the Christ. The calculus for *this* joy is entirely different from our ordinary motives and occasions for celebration. This is joy *in the Lord*. Such joy is truly a gift from God.

This paradoxical, defiant joy also becomes evident in Paul's letter to Philippians when he comments on the mixed motives of those who make the name of Christ known.

> Some proclaim Christ from envy and rivalry, but others from goodwill. These proclaim Christ out of love, knowing that I have been put here for the defense of the gospel; the others proclaim Christ out of selfish ambition, not sincerely but intending to increase my suffering in my imprisonment. What does it matter? Just this, that Christ is proclaimed in every way, whether out of false motives or true; and in that I rejoice. (Phil 1:15–18)

Paul finds joy in that Christ is proclaimed even by those who "proclaim Christ out of selfish ambition, not sincerely but intending to increase my suffering in my imprisonment. What does it matter? Just this, that Christ is proclaimed in every way, whether out of false motives or true; and in that I rejoice." A parallel would be if we were to rejoice even in the behavior of those who intend to hurt us by speaking negatively about our work, because through their bad report, our work becomes more widely known.

Paul gives voice also to this defiant hope in his letter to the Philippians, when he says, "It is by your holding fast to the word of life that I can boast on the day of Christ that I did not run in vain or labor in vain. But even if I am being poured out as a libation over the sacrifice and the offering of your faith, I am glad and rejoice with all of you—and in the same way you also must be glad and rejoice with me" (2:16–18). When Paul speaks here of "being poured out as a libation over the sacrifice," he is alluding to the common ancient sacrificial practice among Jews and pagans of pouring out a portion of wine either over the sacrifice or at the base of the altar in honor to the deity. Paul is the libation and their faith is the sacrifice and offering. It is clear that Paul thinks of what is happening to him in sacrificial terms.[3] Like Peter and the apostles who "rejoiced that they were considered worthy to suffer dishonor for the sake of the name" (Acts 5:41), Paul invites the Philippian Christians to share in this joy defiant of current negative circumstances.

The ground of this sort of joy is God's grace that opens up realities beyond the possibilities of this world. A friend of ours recently gave expression to this defiant joy the day after the funeral of her longtime very close friend. Smiling, several times she said, "I'm not sad, because I know he's in a better place."

The customary ground of joy is some positive circumstance within our life and experience. In my own case, there are many positive circumstances to be joyful about. After more than fifty years of marriage, I still love my wife, Marion, and she still loves me. We have three children, three grandchildren, and in-laws that we love. Marion and I are lucky in that the circumstances of our life are quite good.

Although many circumstances in our life are occasions for joy, other factors are grounds for sorrow. Most prominent is Marion's Alzheimer's disease. The truth is that I am losing my best friend gradually. I am fortunate that this loss is occurring late in our life together, rather than in an

---

3. Scholars differ on *what* Paul's sacrifice is at this point in his life. Some scholars think it refers to his imminent death, even though in just a few sentences later when he speaks of hoping to send Timothy to them, Paul adds, "I trust in the Lord that I will also come soon" (2:24). In any case, Paul is in prison, hardly a happy situation given the wretched state of an ancient prison. It is likely then that Paul considers his strenuous, risky service as an apostle currently in prison as his sacrifice to God. It is in this *sacrificial service* that he takes joy. The point relevant to our concerns is that Paul summons the Philippian Christians to share in this joy.

## JOY

early or middle stage, as happens to some. Nonetheless, the experience of loss for me is real, powerful, and ongoing.

What about Marion's experience? At this point in time, I am unable to describe in any depth Marion's own experience of the disease. From the start, she has been amazingly clear-eyed about it. I no longer ask Marion how she *feels* about having Alzheimer's, because answering that question requires a level of cognitive ability that is now beyond her. In any event, she does not mope or lash out at me or anyone else. She is amazingly cheerful and very appreciative of me.

Long-term progressive dementia gradually squeezes joy out of life. Along the way, though, there may be glimmers of joy. One such glimmer came in an email exchange that I had in November 2018 with a member of Marion's contemplative Mary Circle:

> J: "Hi Brad: Sorry to have missed you yesterday. Marion was very involved in circle yesterday. It was so good to have her thoughtful, prayerful input again."
>
> Brad: "Thanks for the report about Marion. Can you describe her involvement more fully—her 'thoughtful, prayerful input?' I'd appreciate some specifics."
>
> J: "Sure. She found and read her first reading well with just a reminder to keep going. She did read the wrong Bible verse when sharing later, but was able to comment successfully on the positive aspect of the message. In general, her affect was more alert, and Joyce noticed she told Joyce where to turn when returning home. It was a much smaller group and a more traditional Mary Circle, which may have helped. Less chatting, fussing over who will read, etc. Jane kept everyone on task gently. Some of the circle meetings have been more like a traditional Bible study with lots of chatter which, by the way, I also don't appreciate. Marion and I are fives on the enneagram and prefer things quieter and more orderly.
>
> Marion also gave me clear and accurate feedback to my sharing, which was like the old Marion.
>
> I do miss her as I'm sure you must too. J.

The underlying reality, however, is that all such circumstantial occasions for joy will be taken away, maybe tomorrow, but certainly within a few years. This is true both for the one with dementia and those of us who are caregivers. The crucial issue is the source of our joyful experience.

Ordinarily we feel joy when some circumstance turns out well for us. We succeed in a significant endeavor. We get the raise or promotion that we sought. Our loved one recovers from illness. Our son or daughter achieves a worthy goal. Our team wins. Our loved one gives us a hug. In such cases a positive experience is the source of joy. With dementia, though, all usual positive experiences eventually cease.

Since those receiving long-term caregiving are commonly on an extended decline that diminishes their opportunities for experiencing joy, it is vital for those of us who are caregivers to provide them as many occasions for pleasure and joy as possible. Offering opportunities for experiencing joy is a crucial aspect of our ministry.

Music is one vital avenue to joy for many undergoing memory loss. I recall visiting an elderly woman from our congregation named Flo, who was in the memory care unit of a local nursing home. Flo was no longer able to carry on much of a conversation, but she delighted in playing the piano in the common room of the memory unit and with a broad smile singing one of her familiar songs. As someone who for many years had given piano lessons to kids in her home, Flo was a more accomplished musician than most of us, yet music also touches the heart of many who cannot read music or play an instrument.

I must confess, though, that the further Marion declines, the more this message of defiant joy in the face of death becomes a challenge for me. I understand cognitively that the ground for such defiant joy for us Christians is the proclamation of Jesus' resurrection from the dead. I realize that many other people with different religious or philosophical perspectives also affirm some sort of life after death. But life after death is an issue not to be settled by majority vote. It is a question of truth or falsehood that is not answered with the evidence used in ordinary issues of fact. To be sure, death is always near at every point in our life even though we may not feel it. But when one senses death being close at hand for a dear loved one or oneself, the issue is no longer just an intriguing topic to reflect upon or discuss. This is harsh reality. How may I feel *joy* in this situation?

Finding joy in a caregiving situation in which decline is clearly apparent and death lies just over the horizon is a challenge. For those of us doing such caregiving, joy may be in short supply. There may be times in which we do not *feel* any joy. Then the best we can do is to *will* to find joy in God's promises of new life beyond suffering and death. Finally, perhaps that is the best we can do is to find peace for our loved one and ourselves.

CHAPTER FIVE

# Peace

THE APOSTLE PAUL, A Greek-speaking Jew, understood peace, Greek *eirene*, against the background of the Hebrew word *shalom* in the Old Testament. *Shalom* is not just the absence of war between nations or the absence of conflict between individuals or groups. *Shalom* is comprehensive, *positive* unity and well-being. This biblical understanding of peace means wholeness in which divisions are overcome and the community or the various dimensions of an individual person's life function fully and harmoniously. *Shalom* is personal and corporate concord.

It is striking that the apostle Paul speaks of peace in his letter to the Galatians, while in the same letter he carries on a heated controversy with the Jewish Christian missionaries and their supporters who have urged the Galatian Christians to add circumcision to faith in Christ. So the peace of which Paul speaks is not a calm bought at any price, a placid state that overlooks fundamental conflicts. For Paul and the Old Testament tradition, genuine peace is a gift from God in which conflicting factors are overcome or reconciled.

What does it mean to seek this positive peace in a caregiving situation? There are three broad dimensions of peace in the caregiving situation: peace for the one receiving care (both external and internal), peace within the mind and heart of the caregiver, and peace within their family.

## Peace for the One Receiving Care

*1. Safety.* Major personal and social alterations often produce feelings of insecurity in those with dementia. In our case I think Marion and I should stay in our own house as long as possible, for there she is surrounded daily by familiar objects and perspectives; there she feels secure. In our own house, as of summer 2019 she is also able to perform some familiar tasks. Although she is now unable to run our dishwasher, she routinely washes dishes by hand, and on Fridays she still does the laundry and ironing, albeit with occasional assistance from me on operating the washing machine. With some direction from me, in our yard she also is still able to weed, trim plants, rake leaves, and shovel snow.

An extremely important aspect of security for anyone with dementia is personal safety. Safety is an especially crucial concern for those with Parkinson's disease, since the disease attacks the ability to maintain balance. Those with Parkinson's are particularly liable to fall. The wife of a man with Parkinson's hired a woman a few hours a week ostensibly to do some household chores, but the hired woman's chief purpose was to be at home with him while the wife ran some errands.

The son of a father with Parkinson's and mother with Alzheimer's made this comment about his parents' move from their hometown house to a care facility near the son:

> It was a matter of safety. In fact, the precipitating event was a pretty serious fall. My father had fallen outside, and my mother didn't remember that he was outside. He was finally able to get back into the house. She just didn't know that he was in such an extreme situation. If he hadn't been able to return. . . . That experience frightened us all, and I think it was a wake-up call for him, that yes, I need to be in an assisted living situation.

On several occasions during the night a wife, whose husband had Parkinson's, found him lying on the floor somewhere in their house. When she was unable to get him up, she had to call for help. Although he had not fallen in this instance, his difficulty maintaining balance meant that he was vulnerable to falling in the future. The danger of a serious injury was real.

Safety concerns arise in dealing with other forms of dementia as well. I worry some that with her Alzheimer's, Marion might get stranded on our deck, which has no stairs to the ground eight feet below. If she were stranded on the deck, especially on a very hot or very cold day, she might injure herself trying to drop to the ground. Consequently, before I leave home, I routinely check that our kitchen door to the deck is unlocked. However, in June 2019, a new wrinkle took me by surprise. While I was away for two days on a personal retreat, our daughter Julie stayed with Marion. On the second afternoon of her stay, Julie and Marion became trapped on our deck, because the storm/screen door to the deck became locked. After about three hours of their slapping away mosquitoes and yelling for help, Julie was finally heard shouting by the son of our neighbor across the street, who has a key to our house. The son gained entrance to our house and opened the door to the deck.

Finding the right balance between giving Marion space and keeping her safe is sometimes difficult. I discovered this with Marion's afternoon visit to her friend Ag in early October 2018. When we arrived in the parking lot of the assisted living complex where Ag lives now, Marion said that I should not come in with her. I agreed, because when I am present, the extroverted Ag tends to talk more with me than with introverted Marion. I told Marion that Ag had her name on her apartment door. So I waited in our car for several minutes, and then went inside to check on things. Ag's name was no longer on her door. When I knocked and went in, Ag was alone. So I searched for Marion, and finally located her in a section of the attached nursing home; she had been unable to find Ag's apartment. We went to Ag's unit, and I told them I would come back in about an hour. When I returned, Ag was alone; Marion had left. After searching fruitlessly through the main portions of the nursing home, I drove on streets that I thought Marion would likely take to get home. No sight of her. So I headed for home, thinking that I might have to call the police for assistance. As I turned onto our street, I saw in my rearview mirror Marion walking on the edge of the Luther College campus and headed toward home. When she got into the car, she was calm. I was far less so. When I reported this incident to our daughter Julie, she said, "Mom's sense of direction is still very good. When I was with her, she told me just where to go." However, this incident has made me more cautious about leaving Marion on her own in our town. She does fine when she goes out for a solo walk in our immediate neighborhood, but I feel I must be careful when she goes beyond that.

2. *Inner peace.* Another dimension of peace in caregiving is internal, peace within the person receiving care. Of course, a fundamental goal in any caregiving situation is to have the recipient of care feel at peace. This involves a sense of not only being safe, but also valued. I am confident that, on the whole, in our home situation Marion does feel both safe and valued. Living with me in our house since 1990 gives her stability, security, and the assurance of being loved. So, while it must be unsettling for her to feel somewhat adrift in a wider environment that she understands less and less, there is

security and peace in her immediate, familiar physical and social world. Indeed, in the summer of 2018 when we left that familiar context and flew to Los Angeles for a week visiting our younger son and grandson and then flew to Seattle for five days with her sister Elaine, as we got ready for bed on the first evening of both visits, she asked me, "Are we going home tomorrow?" At the time, I thought this came merely from her inability to keep track of time, but now I see it mainly as her yearning to be in a familiar context.

Peace within the loved one receiving care is not within the full control of the caregiver, yet it is very important how the caregiver responds to unsettling factors in the environment and within the loved one. Peace within the one receiving care will vary depending in great measure on the person's stage of dementia—early, middle, or late stage.

*Early stage*: Our loved one may not be able to articulate the concern, but it may be manifest in his or her behavior. For example, in an interview this husband, whose wife developed Alzheimer's disease, expressed how he gradually realized that his wife's unrest precipitated some significant changes in their life together.

> My wife and I are quite different, independent people. We have a lovely house, a big house. I have my library, a television, and books; everything I want. And she has her place in the kitchen and the TV there. She's a sports fanatic, and she loves to watch sports on TV. I couldn't care less. I enjoy the computer, theology, and history. We read different things, have different interests. We're just very different people when it comes to entertainment.

*Peace within the recipient of care as the disease advances.* The feeling of insecurity may increase as the disease advances. While Marion has not exhibited feelings of physical insecurity, she does manifest feelings of what I may call social insecurity. For example, on a September 2018 morning Marion was trying to select clothes appropriate for a three-day trip we were going to begin later that day. The occasion for the trip was to attend the funeral of my sister's husband, but I had also arranged to visit Marion's brother and his wife before the funeral and visit an old childhood friend after the funeral. Because Marion was aware that we were going away sometime in the near future, but did not grasp the time interval, she had already started to pack for the trip three days in advance. So, after her breakfast on the day of our midday departure, I was surprised to find that she had unpacked her suitcase and was trying on one outfit after another. Several pairs of slacks no longer fit her, since within the last year she had uncharacteristically gained about fifteen pounds. In addition, she was having difficulty distinguishing between her need for casual clothes for the majority of our time away and more formal dress for the funeral. I tried to help by bringing forward different possibilities. I must admit that I became a little irritated with going around and around. But I tried to curb my irritation and be calm. After she settled finally on an outfit for the funeral, I soon left for a couple hours at my office. However, I realized that she might well go through the search again later in the morning.

*Peace within the recipient of care during a late stage*: A woman whose father has died and whose mother is in the final stage of Lewy body dementia commented:

> Now my mom's mental character for much of the day is like a three-year-old's. Now she is really like a child. The other day she had a teddy bear, and it was wrapped in a towel like a blanket, and she was singing childhood songs and church hymns to her. She is really very child-like. I do feel like her parent in some ways. That means that in a lot of ways, I don't have a mom. Recently, I had a bad cold and didn't visit her for a couple days. I remember being overwhelmed, just needing to tell her, "Mom, I wasn't feeling well." When I was able to visit her again, she put her hand on my leg and said, "You just need to get more rest." That was a very motherly thing to say, and it felt really good, *really* good. Yah.

## Peace within the Caregiver

The second broad dimension of peace in caregiving is peace within the caregiver. A vital aspect of this is the caregiver's personal peace with his or her role as caregiver. Having peace in one's caregiving role has several aspects.

1. *One absolutely vital and fundamental aspect is full-hearted commitment to caregiving this particular person needing care.*

It may take some time to arrive at full-hearted commitment as we adjust to a new, very different situation. The disability or dementia may develop for some time without being recognized, even if one is living with the person from day to day. As C, an old friend and physician married for over fifty years, said in a phone interview from his spacious oceanside home:

> We've had a great marriage. Then things changed. Two or three years ago, for example, she wanted to learn about the computer. Each time, it was as though she was there for the first time. I'd get very angry. I'd leave, throwing up my hands. And she'd leave the same. A medical examination revealed that she had some treatable medical conditions—deficits of B12 vitamin and folic acid. There is no question that having treated these over the last year, her neurological confusion has cleared. And basically, what we're left with is an individual with virtually no short-term memory. So I don't tell her about what we'll do in three days, because she'll ask me forty times about it before it happens. More importantly, I realize that my frustration and anger early on were coming from an understanding that was not accurate.
>
> But change came. She no longer wanted me out of the kitchen. She wanted me not only on *my* side of the couch [in the everyday family dining area], but she wanted me to be physically in the room on *her* side of the couch. I got the feeling that she wanted me, physically, in her room. That required an adjustment. This interrupted my way of being in the house.
>
> Emotionally, I think there was a questioning on her part about my love and devotion to her. I think she was anxious about that. She was implicitly asking, "Do you love me?" She was aware that there was something driving me away. And I'm not sure that she wasn't correct. In other words, she was aware that there was something in *her* driving me away, something in her. It was a real question of my love and devotion for her.
>
> She was very acute in feeling something was not right anymore. And that anger surfaced enough so that she suspicioned and felt there was something going on. This lasted six months. I've come to realize that there was something to that. . . . But at the same time, I have *never, ever* felt I wanted to dump the situation. She has been my life. And I told her this morning [voice breaks], when I see her, I see the person who knows more about me and knows what we've been through over the last sixty years. And I think she is coming to an understanding and being comfortable in that. She no longer sees that as a threat.

Generally, I believe Marion also feels valued and loved by me. We hug and kiss frequently throughout the day. However, her sense of being loved by me is fragile, for from time to time she asks me, "Are you mad at me?"

Usually this takes me by surprise, and I immediately reassure her that I love her. Yet I suspect that this occurs when she feels that I am emotionally distant from her. Although I do not truly get angry with her personally, from time to time I get tired and emotionally withdraw for awhile.

Others doing caregiving in their home found some relief by hiring someone to come in for a few hours a week a relief. The motives for doing this included both easing strain on the caregiver and guarding the safety of the one receiving care. As one woman commented on caring for her husband with Parkinson's disease:

> About a year before he went to the nursing home, it was clear that it had become more unsafe for him to be alone. So I became more uncomfortable leaving him alone even for short periods of time. And it was difficult to ask if it was OK for me to leave him home alone, because I didn't want him to feel I didn't trust him. So initially . . . after quite a bit of thought, I engaged a woman who worked here in this building doing various odd jobs for tenants. Just at the beginning I asked her to be here for an hour or so, so I could go out and do some errands. So she came and without being obvious about it, did some cleaning and household things, but she was clearly here to make it safe for him. And it made it possible for me to get some time out. She came a couple times a week for probably a year.

If we are pulled unwillingly into the role of caregiver by circumstances such as being the family member geographically closest, we may resent this burden and resent the one needing care as well as other family members who are less able or less willing to help. Indeed, full-hearted commitment to caregiving this person may not be our initial response. If a loved one has a gradual decline, we may have time to adjust little by little to the new situation. But sometimes circumstances change rapidly, and we do not have the opportunity to sort out our feelings and priorities. The responsibility is thrust upon us, and we are left with the task of sifting through our feelings and motives while carrying out these unsought responsibilities. In such a case it may take time to resolve our conflicting concerns. Talking with a trusted person may assist in this process.

It may be that our relationship with the one needing care has a rocky history. For instance, author Jade Angelica tells of her very conflicted history with her mother. Jade and her mother had been separated geographically and emotionally for more than twenty years. Jade lived in Maine and her mother lived in Iowa. But more significantly for a long time Jade had separated herself from her mother's alcoholic lifestyle and judgmental nature. Jade continued to avoid her mother even after she learned from a cousin that her mom, like several other family members before, was showing signs of dementia. Their relationship took a turn for the better when this cousin brought Jade's mother to Maine for a visit. Jade was surprised to find that her mother's judgmental attitude had been replaced with a kind of sweetness. Jade ended up moving back to Iowa, and taking care of her mother until her mother's death.[1]

Even if one is willing to be the primary caregiver, taking on that role is likely to exact a price that is not clearly understood from the beginning. Becoming the primary caregiver requires changes in one's own life, and affects how much time and energy one can devote to other cherished activities or relationships. For example, the favorite pastime of a husband whose wife developed dementia was fly fishing. While at first he thought he would have to give up his fishing hobby, in a phone interview a bit later he planned to adjust his fishing practice to the new circumstances.

> You realize that your life has changed. Before, I'd go off for a week four or five times a year to North Carolina for fishing, but I can't do that anymore. I realize that the next phase of my trout fishing, that's been going on over the last thirty years in various parts of the country, is basically over. So my hobby, which is basically fishing, is really over. . . . And adjusting to that . . . I was getting tired of fishing anyway [laugh]. That's part defense mechanism, I'm sure [laugh], but she can't do that anymore. Fishing has been my hobby. Adjusting to that, anyway.
>
> So I'll take her with me. Unfortunately, when I take her along to North Carolina with me, I can't take a cheap $52 motel, but have to spend $75 for one on the water. So I've solved that by taking her with me, and showing her my "girlfriends" at the waffle place and then having a nice dinner at the casino. So I've solved that by taking her with me. So not worrying about her at home and wondering whether people, who are supposed to show up, do show up. Or worrying about her falling at night, which she has done a few times when I've been here. So I've solved that by taking her with me. This gives me some future. Whereas six months ago, from that standpoint, I had no future. This gives some future.

---

1. Angelica, *Where Two Worlds Touch: A Spiritual Journey Through Alzheimer's Disease* (Boston: Skinner House, 2014), 5–14.

However, his wife's condition worsened to the point that this modified plan also had to be abandoned. In its place, though, family members came to his rescue, as he reported in this email:

> Good to hear from you, Brad, and happy that the medical status in your house is stable. Your comments on help with Marion while you were away struck a note with me: our three girls were here for [my wife's] birthday 12/22 and we arranged for them to pitch in with her care a week in April, whilst I go fishing up in NC ending my two-year fishing drought up there. They've always said they'd be available and I'm cashing some of those chips in!
>
> Also I'm making a move to find out what help the local Alzheimer Association can provide for us. I've not done anything in that regard yet and finally feel I should; e.g., a local Methodist church has a four-hour session twice a week with activities and lunch provided. We'll see.
>
> As to her current condition, she has no short-term memory, now sleeping more hours and is a bit more contentious than before. She's at that sorrowful stage of knowing her problem, knowing there's no cure, wondering how fast it's going to progress. She's always wanting to go back to "our other house," doesn't know her way around this house we've lived eighteen years in. Otherwise she's very healthy celebrating her eighty-second BDay recently. I'm fine presently, but recognizing we should get some help before we need some help. We're coping . . . and I'm becoming a damn fine cook . . . anybody for Chicken Francaise ( . . . the $6.00 lunch is just called chicken French). Enough for now. Good '19 wishes.

Some caregivers are fortunate to start out with some habitual practices that foster emotional closeness with the one needing care. Marion and I have several such practices: having a hug and kiss just before I leave for my office, having afternoon tea together, taking a late afternoon walk together, and touching hands while saying "I love you" before we go to sleep. One woman who cared at home for her husband with Parkinson's said, "Strangely, the closest we were on any given day was when we went to bed at night. We'd say the Creed together, and he might be struck by something, and would stop and discourse on something that rang a bell to him. And then we'd say the Lord's Prayer and go to sleep. Those were close times."

Taking on primary responsibility for care may be complicated by an emotional burden that one already is bearing. This middle-aged woman has primary responsibility for her elderly mother after her father has died. She said,

> I would say that another challenge for me is the grief that I carry for my twenty-year-old son, who died almost five years ago. It's a challenge walking together with her with that trunk of grief already attached to my hip. I talked with a counselor a month ago, how losing her will be so different than losing Dad. Suddenly, it hit me: I'm like her parent now. So in many ways, I'm getting ready to lose another child. And that is really hard. *Really hard.*

Even if we willingly take on caregiving, its stresses over time put an enormous strain on our body and spirit. When speaking with my wife, I am much more likely to have an edge to my voice when I am tired. Fatigue is fertile soil for irritability, and irritability tends to produce sharp words and unkind actions.

*2. Factors Contributing to a Caregiver's Fatigue and Irritability*
I have found that an increase of irritability within me is closely correlated with growing fatigue. Sometimes my fatigue is directly connected with sleeping poorly, but other times, even when I have been sleeping well, after several weeks I feel fatigue creeping up on me.

Several factors in a long-term, home caregiving situation may contribute to fatigue. One factor may be that caregiving Dad or Mom or our spouse comes on top of *a high level of pre-existing caregiving responsibility.* This has not been the case for me personally, since our three children are self-supporting adults and our parents are deceased. But some caregivers of an elderly parent already have responsibility for another elderly person or still have children at home for whom they must care. For instance, one mother caring for her mother had several children of various ages at home, and misunderstandings and conflicts sometimes arose between the grandmother and the children.

> At first Mom lived across the street from us in her own little house. We sent kids over with her meds. She had some anger issues; she said, "Someone called the police on me." It was ugly.
>
> In 2012 we moved to a lot smaller town. Now she lived with us. It was no longer safe for her to be on her own. She had a gas stove and might not remember to turn off the propane. Enough things could go wrong; it was no longer safe. So she came to live with us.
>
> That was definitely the hardest phase for me. She had some anger issues. She was angry about a dog across the street. She had some hallucinations. With us, she wasn't keeping house much

anymore. Before, when she was alone, she walked her dog, but by the time she came with us, she almost never left the house. We had some conflicts between her and our kids. That was the hardest part on me. I felt like I was between Mom and my kids. They understood, but it was hard trying to explain things to them. That part was hardest on me. Sometimes Mom was pretty hateful to our kids. We had two daughters—one with brown hair and one with blond. And she got them confused. One day, our son cut his hand and later that day she freaked out. Mom yelled at the kids. *Her understanding* of it was that our son was married to "a blond floozy." There was a lot of that stuff with her. It got to be a lot. Then my sisters stepped in and pushed to have Mom in a facility.

A second factor increasing fatigue is a *gradual reduction in variety*. For much of our adult life, many of us can get away from the stress of our daily work by taking a vacation, often going away to a different place for awhile. The husband who loves to flyfish has found his favorite pastime limited by caregiving his wife. When Marion and I were both working, we always went away for a week or two, most often camping, but sometimes taking a long trip to visit family on the west coast. Since we both retired, we have spent four to six weeks almost every winter in Houston, Texas. The fresh personal relationships, interesting Southern culture, easy access to a great opera, symphony, and art museums made these visits stimulating. A major difficulty with long-term caregiving is that variety gradually gets squeezed out, and there is much less spice in life. For Marion and me it is unlikely that we will ever again spend a few weeks in Houston.

A third major factor contributing to fatigue in caregiving a loved one is the *feeling that in some sense one is always on call*. In my case, with Marion in the second stage of Alzheimer's, I am still able to leave her on her own when I go every weekday morning to my college library office. I return home for lunch and a short nap. Return to my office for part of the afternoon has ceased for the most part as I move further into my eighties. Of course, when I'm in my office, I'm just a phone call and five-minute trip away. But I expect that at some point, it will no longer be safe for me to leave her at home alone for a few hours. So, on the one hand, I appreciate the relative freedom I have currently. On the other hand, even when I'm in town away from home, I always have the feeling of being on call.

The most restful time for me happens when one of our three children comes to stay with Marion, and I go away for a forty-eight-hour private retreat. Nevertheless, even when I am away on retreat, I am always aware of Marion. In the back of my mind is always the possibility that I might be called home early. Indeed, after about twenty hours away on retreat, I always call home just to check how Marion is doing. To be sure, I do not resent Marion. I do not in the least feel that she is a burdensome weight around my neck. In fact, I feel it is a gift and privilege for me to care for her. Some people lose a dear loved one in a moment or a few days. Marion and I have the opportunity to share this part of our married life together for an extended period of time. Nevertheless, I always feel that I am on call.

The feeling of being on call is common with family caregivers. When I interviewed an elderly woman who cared for her husband with memory loss from diminished blood supply to the brain ("vascular cognitive impairment"). I asked, What were the major challenges that she experienced in caregiving? She answered,

> I would say not having *any* time to myself. It was like after we would go to bed at night, I would get up and go into the TV room and sit and read for a little while. Then after it seemed like two or three minutes, he'd be in there asking, "Aren't you coming to bed?" I'd say, "Soon." Then after five minutes, he'd come and say, "Aren't you coming to bed?" So finally, I'd give up and go to bed.
>
> Another thing. I'd come and say, "I'm going into the bathroom now, and I'm going to take a bath. Is that OK?" He'd say, "Sure." I'd hardly be in there a minute, and he'd say, "Are you OK?" Then in just a few minutes, he'd be asking, "Aren't you done yet?" That sort of thing became for me the most . . . I have another friend who says the same thing—the need to just let your mind go and relax a little.

A woman in her early sixties said this about caregiving her ninety-plus mother, "It's been very rewarding sometimes. Sometimes it tries my patience."

I responded, "You say it tries your patience. How do you cope with that?"

She answered:

> Well, at times I put myself in a time-out. If I feel I'm going in that direction, I will go into the bathroom and have a few minutes to myself.
>
> I have a friend back home with six kids; she would run herself ragged and her health would take a hit. I told her, "You've got to keep yourself fit. If that well of yours runs dry, you don't have anything to run on." I have to remember that myself. Sometimes I just need to get out of the house, go for a walk, do some gardening. . . .

> That whole patience thing is challenging. Sometimes I'd take a time-out. I'd go upstairs; she doesn't go there anymore, and I'd say, "I need a time-out."

Some home caregivers have more opportunity to find alone time. One wife first identified traveling as a major challenge in caregiving, but then secondly, she added, "Insisting on my own space and quiet time. I'm usually able to manage that. I stay up at night."

I asked, "He's OK with that?"

She replied, "Typically he goes to bed early, by eight. Sometimes he comes back down and he interrupts 'my quiet time'—and that's OK. So, it's not necessarily an external quiet, but internal."

So, one of the common challenges of family caregiving is coming to terms with the feeling that one is always on call, of finding some way to truly relax.

A fourth factor adding to a family caregiver's fatigue may be *the progressive accumulation of grief*. In my case, I am *little by little losing my dearest friend*. To watch Marion very gradually diminish in her abilities is heartbreaking for me. When a loved one dies, we have external expressions of grief that are socially supported and approved. Crying, wailing, sitting vigil are common, outward, and socially accepted ways of dealing with a loved one's death. But how does one express grief for a loved one's gradual diminishment over a number of years? I suspect that only those who have themselves experienced this can understand and give support. Whereas joy is energizing, grieving drains us of vitality.

A fifth factor fostering fatigue for us older caregivers is *the gradual loss of other good friends, so that we have less social support from people who know us well*. Now that I am in my mid-eighties, I have lost a number of good friends. I have previously told the story of losing a good friend, Paul, to colon cancer. Paul's absence left a hole in my life, because I had now lost the one male friend with whom I could share most fully my feelings about caregiving.

A sixth factor adding to my fatigue is that Marion's *diminishing interaction with and support from her friends increases her reliance on me*. Friendships are built and sustained by mutual sharing, which takes place on several levels. A basic level of sharing occurs by participating in an activity done in common with another individual or a group. Deeper levels of sharing require fuller engagement of personal thought and emotion through verbal and non-verbal communication. Among Marion's shared activities over the last several decades, those that had high priority for her have been the monthly meeting of her contemplative church women's group, the Mary Circle, and the monthly gathering of women knitting prayer shawls. During our winter weeks in Houston, she treasured meeting twice a week with a small group of women for morning prayer. Especially prized by her were opportunities for using her gifts and training as a spiritual director with the two-year Spiritual Formation Program of Grace Institute for Spiritual Formation and with individuals who came to our home for periodic visits. Also important as purely social gatherings have been the weekly afternoon coffee time with the women in the Menders and the May-through-September weekly couples' picnic supper in a park.

The last ten to twelve years have brought the gradual diminishment of Marion's involvement in these corporate activities, and consequently a steady reduction of her social interactions and the gradual drying up of friendships. Since she is less and less able to carry on a conversation, she becomes more and more socially isolated. So, when summer 2019 arrived, we had to decide what to do about the weekly Wednesday evening picnic supper in a park that we had participated in for more than twenty years. I raised the issue of attending the picnic with Marion, and she was noncommittal. Although I enjoy the conversations at these informal events, her social isolation makes me wonder whether we should stop going. The previous summer I noticed that Marion was not the only one socially isolated, for I observed that another woman with dementia also stood off by herself, not engaged in conversation with others. I decided that we would not attend the picnic. Given her reduction in social engagement, Marion and I especially appreciate members of her weekly Menders group and monthly Mary Circle who have been amazingly faithful in contacting her about meeting time and place, and helping her get to their gatherings. Nevertheless, the harsh reality of dementia is that even while Marion is physically present with another individual or group, she has less and less *personal presence.*

This unavoidable diminishment of Marion's social support makes my presence and support absolutely critical for her well-being. I spend by far the most time with her. Fortunately, Marion and I are best friends, and as wife and husband we enjoy expressing our love and support with frequent hugs, kisses, touching of hands, warm shared smiles, and sex now and then. As I reflect on this, it dawns on me that never before have I been so profoundly needed by anyone.

## 3. The Caregiver's Vocation to Provide Security and Love

The circumstances of my shared life with Marion have thrust upon me the most far-reaching and difficult *vocation* of my life. The concept of vocation, derived from the Latin word for calling, was given deep, comprehensive significance by Martin Luther and other Protestant Reformers. Prior to Luther the idea of vocation was commonly limited to those who accepted a religious calling to the priesthood or life in a religious order, such as the Benedictine order of men and women. The Protestant Reformers taught that every person is given a vocation, indeed multiple vocations. For example, for many years I was called to be a professor, a husband to Marion, a father to our three children, a son to my parents, and a citizen in a democratic society. Fulfilling these social roles has given me multiple vocations. Now as Marion's cognitive capabilities decline my calling as her husband takes on greater depth: I am especially called to help her feel secure and loved.

In addition to fostering stability for Marion, I am called to help her feel valued and loved even as other social signs of worth, affection, and esteem diminish. Fortunately, I do not need to work at this or deliberately follow some printed list of kindly actions. I love her and, above all else, I want her to feel appreciated and loved. As I realize this dimension of my responsibility toward her, I also grow in appreciation for those family members, friends, and professional caregivers who render stable, kind assistance to persons who are difficult, unappreciative, or even hostile toward them.

While walking alone in our neighborhood one June 2018 afternoon, it dawned on me that caregiving Marion is a gift. It's not a gift in the usual sense of something we have desired and are gleeful about receiving. It is gift in a more subtle way. On the one hand, I think of those who lose a loved one suddenly with no opportunity to say thank you and goodbye. At least my losing of Marion and her losing of me and all that she loves take place gradually. We have time to hold hands, hug, and kiss. We have time to say thank you to one another. Our children have time to hug and thank their mom. On the other hand, caregiving Marion is also a gift for me in the sense that a calling can be a gift. My calling in the work place was to be a professor of religion. While I enjoyed and loved the work, I also felt that what I did was meaningful to others, or at least could be meaningful. Objectively, my work gave me the opportunity to assist young adults in thinking through some fundamental questions of human existence. Subjectively, I also had a sense that my work as a teacher was appreciated by quite a few of my students. My calling to care for Marion is a gift in similar fashion. While I do rather enjoy cooking and finding a recipe that we like, far more significant is the reality that caregiving Marion is deeply meaningful, probably the most significant activity of my life. There is nothing more important for me now than helping her feel safe and loved.

*4. Ways for A Caregiver to Replenish Inner Peace and Generous Love*
If we are to continue long-term as a caregiver, we need to find ways to refresh our spirit by letting go of resentments and replenishing generous love. The ways of replenishment will vary with a person's interests and experience, but they are likely near at hand.

One woman caring for her mother, who is in a care center, said that what keeps her on track is her daily devotional practice of reading Scripture, doing centering prayer, and writing in her journal.

In addition to his daily practice of prayer, a male pastor caring for one parent with Alzheimer's and the other parent with Parkinson's said, "A major resource for me has been the life experience as a pastor with families who have gone through the stages of a family member with these two diseases. I see others who don't know what's ahead, but I do, since I've walked this road."

When I asked another woman, "What resources or help (if any) have you found in your caregiving?" She replied,

> I've done a kind of mental spread sheet of the remarkable women I've known in my life, beginning with both of my grandmothers, who were immigrants and struggled. My mother's mother came to this country, had six kids, five sons who went off to war and all came back. My father's mother raised not only her kids, but also her brother-in-law's kids because his wife was in a mental institution. There were thirteen kids in a little bitty house. And all of those kids did OK. My mother and my sister. And now I think of my sister-in-law, who is exhausted almost every day. And one of our dear friends in Wisconsin, who is frail and cares for her husband, who is very difficult, very difficult. And the women in my church circle. Think of these women! Just remarkable women! I hear my Russian grandmother with all the trials and tribulations she had; she was very fatalistic. All the women in my life. Just deal with it. Just deal with it. Get over it. So . . . I can hear them talking.

This woman also relied on her regular practice of crafting. She said, "I'll show you how grace is shed on us—one of the ways grace is shed is crafting. This [holding up a piece] is crochet, but I knit too. And I encourage him [her husband] to do his craft. He has always liked to work in wood, and I've encouraged him to do that."

I asked, "What is it about knitting and crocheting that is beneficial for you?"

> Well, for the most part, it's doing something to give away. All of these [various knitted and crocheted objects] are gifts. We have taken classes in crafting, and if they work—they haven't always worked—but if they work, then we've had gifts to give away at Christmas time. I've done spoons, Hardanger embroidery.[2] I'll show you my latest fascination. It's a little octopus. . . . Here is Elmer the Elephant; he went to our nephew's son. So anyway, that's worth a lot.
>
> The gifts go with poems, so I wrote silly poems to go with the gifts. And I get a big kick out of all of that.

Her comment triggered this response in me:

> All of us caregivers would do well to ask, "What do I get a big kick out of?"

*5. Personally, I have found four practices that together reduce my irritability and fortify my inner peace: swearing, physical activity, daily meditation, and periodic private retreat.*

### a. Swearing

The quickest and most at hand way to reduce my irritability is to let off steam by swearing. For many years, I had used crude or off-color language very sparingly. But since I've been caregiving with Marion, I say "shit" or "son of a bitch" much more often. It's not something I plan. It just comes out in the moment. Publicly, I don't swear out loud, but in some situations I swear under my breath.

Although for many years I had seldom swore, I noticed that as my caregiving responsibilities with Marion gradually increased, so did the frequency of my swearing. I have not beat myself up about it, because I sense that the practice is beneficial to Marion and to me. Swearing alerts me to

---

2. Hardanger embroidery is a form of embroidery traditionally worked with white thread on white even-weave linen or cloth, using counted thread and drawn thread work techniques that flourished in the Hardanger area of Norway from 1650 to 1850.

the fact that I am feeling stressed. More importantly, it has felt to me that swearing helps relieve my stress. It's like a safety valve that lowers pressure within me.

I can tell that I'm getting very fatigued if I say, "God dammit," because I've always been very careful about not using God's name in vain, and I have scrupulously avoided the trivialization of God's name in the recently popular expressions, "Oh my God" and "OMG." If I were to beat myself up about an occasional "God dammit," it would make my situation worse, and I would become even more irritable and more liable to lash out at Marion. But I have felt that God is generous enough to allow me to release tension even by misusing God's name occasionally.

I have been confirmed in my acceptance of limited swearing by reading British science writer Emma Byrne's 2017 book *Swearing Is Good for You: The Amazing Science of Bad Language*. One striking scientific experiment she cites was done by a British psychologist, Dr. Richard Stephens, with sixty-seven of his male and female undergraduate students. The students were asked to put both their hands in ice cold water for as long as they could stand it. They did this twice. Once without swearing, and once while swearing. Beforehand, the professor asked each student to identify five words they would use if they dropped a hammer on their thumb and five words each would use to describe a neutral object such as a table. Then for the ice water experiment the professor assigned each student the first word in their two lists. So, for example, when holding her hands under the ice cold water, one student might say the neutral word "sturdy" over and over. Then later holding her hands under the ice cold water, this same student would say "shit" over and over. The order in which the students did this was randomized, so that roughly half the students swore during the first trial and half swore during the second trial. Emma Byrne reports,

> It turned out that, when they were swearing, the intrepid volunteers could keep their hands in the water nearly half again as long as when they used their table-based adjectives. Not only that, while they were swearing the volunteers' heart rates went up and their *perception* of pain went down: in other words, the volunteers experienced less pain while swearing.[3]

One might think these benefits of swearing come only to those who are accustomed to expressing their anger. But this is not the case. Professor

---

3. Byrne, *Swearing Is Good for You: The Amazing Science of Bad Language* (New York: W. W. Norton, 2017), 48.

Stephens found that his results held true for both those who tend to express their angry a lot ("anger-out" people) and those who tend to hold their anger in ("anger-in" people). Stephens also found that milder forms of naughty language are not as effective in countering pain as stronger swear words.[4] In my own case, the occasional "God dammit" is then an indication that I am feeling a high level of stress.

Is swearing also effective with other sources of suffering than physical pain? Dr. Sarah Seymour-Smith at the British University of Huddersfield found that swearing was a beneficial way that men with a serious illness such as testicular cancer could deal with their feelings in losing one or both testicles. She tells of one man, dubbed Cal, who would not go to a self-help group to talk about his feelings, but on a privately made video, he used swearing and dark humor to affirm his identity. "He starts by talking about how 'shit' the year has been, and says that it's 'really bollocks, er . . . bollock sorry!'" These men also turned to dark humor. They used words like "womble" (which sounds like "one-ball") or spoke of being a member of the "flatbaggers club." Emma Byrne says, "Dr. Seymour-Smith's research suggests that talking in this taboo-breaking, jokey manner is 'a way of reworking a positive identity from having both testicles removed.' A means of both dealing with the pain and reasserting his masculinity."[5]

Swearing may not have the same positive affect for women with serious illness. Emma Byrne says, "It is far more socially acceptable for women to talk about their feelings, even to cry, but if they vent their emotions with swearing it doesn't go well for them. In a lab, with a bucket of ice, swearing helps women as much as men, but in the real world, with long-term, life-changing pain, women lose out when they swear."[6]

A study by Professor Megan Robbins at the University of Arizona found that women with breast cancer and other long-term serious health conditions who swore around other women ended up more depressed and with less support from friends than those who did not swear. This study recorded a portion of the women's speech over a weekend. When Robbins followed up later with these women, "she found that the women who swore more around their female friends tended to lose those friends over the course of their illness and to end up more depressed."[7]

4. Byrne, *Swearing Is Good for You*, 58.
5. Byrne, *Swearing Is Good for You*, 63.
6. Byrne, *Swearing Is Good for You*, 63.
7. Byrne, *Swearing Is Good for You*, 64.

However, women's readiness to swear is correlated with their age and their cultural context. Older woman, especially those born before 1960, tend to be uncomfortable with swearing. Women swearing is also influenced by their cultural context; it is more common and accepted in the United Kingdom than in Canada and the more religiously conservative United States. Emma Byrne says, "From South Africa to Northern Ireland, Great Britain to the United States, women are judged more harshly than men for swearing. Teenage girls in the 1990s—my contemporaries and the daughters of second-wave feminists—considered swearing to be far less acceptable from a woman than a man, even though women now account for 45 percent of all swearing in public (up from 33 percent in 1986)."[8]

Byrne asks, "Is there really a difference in the *reasons why* men and women swear? There might be. Men tend to feel comfortable using swearing in a jokey manner, as well as using it as a tool. For women, swearing is much more likely to be instrumental, to be used very carefully for effect. Professors Bailey and Timm found that the women they interviewed were also more likely to use swear words as a rhetorical device, to inject a bit of 'punch' into their conversation."[9]

Dr. Karyn Stapleton thinks that women use swearing instrumentally, to make an impression or to be heard in mixed company. However, she says swearing is much more socially risky for women than for men. Stapleton says, "The division of language into purity and power might still be responsible for women's reluctance to swear. 'From numerous studies we know that women are expected to pay more attention to politeness than men. Swearing can be incredibly direct.' Because of the double pressure of inviting moral censure and being judged harshly for failing to be polite, 'choosing to swear is still a much higher risk for women.'"[10]

None of the women I interviewed—most of them senior citizens—*volunteered* that they swore. Rather, two spoke of responding to frustration by having a "melt-down." When I asked one woman who used this term, "What happens in a melt-down?" the following exchange took place:

I said, "What happens to *you*?"
She said, "I have an Italian fit."
I asked, "That means?"
She answered, "I go off and pound the wall."

---

8. Byrne, *Swearing Is Good for You*, 153.
9. Byrne, *Swearing Is Good for You*, 162.
10. Byrne, *Swearing Is Good for You*, 153–54.

"Literally?"

"Sometimes. That's it. Deal with it."

Later when I followed up by email to ask specifically whether she finds swearing to be an outlet for frustration and anger, she very guardedly and in general terms only admitted to swearing, but she also answered insightfully about the risk and limits of swearing in a caregiving relationship: "Indeed, I find swearing useful and even salutary. But it's not helpful in the presence of someone who is fragile. I do my best to keep an even and clean tone in his presence. I do not want him to think he exasperates me (which he sometimes does) or, especially, that he is a burden to me (which he is not)."

After receiving this answer, I followed up with another woman (in her upper eighties) who had said nothing about swearing when I had previously interviewed her. But now when I specifically asked, she too admitted that she swore sometimes during her caregiving years. "You know, it's sort of like when I bump my leg, I say sh . . . " [not finishing the word].

Another woman said, "Sometimes swearing happens—it is not a conscious thing, but can come out in an agitated moment or when I am recounting an agitated moment with my mom to my spouse. It is not, however, a consistent thing for me."

Yet another woman caregiver, whose husband had died, replied, "I don't recall swearing, it's not my thing. I would find it not helpful."

These responses confirmed Emma Byrne's assertion that women's readiness to swear is correlated with their age and their cultural context. Older women, especially those born before 1960, tend to be uncomfortable with swearing. This is certainly true of Marion, because I have never heard her swear even with a mild word. Recently when she was frustrated over something, her verbal response was a hearty, "Bummer."

Those doing research on swearing distinguish two distinct types of swearing: *propositional swearing* and *non-propositional swearing*. Byrne says, "Propositional swearing is deliberately chosen for effect," whereas non-propositional swearing "is the unplanned, unintended outburst that comes when we're surprised or hurt, and draws more heavily on the emotion-processing parts of the brain."[11] So the use of a swear word as I and other caregivers vent our frustration with the burdens of caregiving or as those students held their hands under ice water is non-propositional use of swearing. It is a venting of emotion.

---

11. Byrne, *Swearing Is Good for You*, 17.

Propositional swearing is done intentionally for social effect. Very common today in the United States is the use of swearing to express deep disagreement with a political party or leader with whom we strongly disagree. The addition of swear words intensifies one's disagreement. Swearing verbally is like the use of italics or underlining in written communication with the addition of strong emotional coloring.

In my case as an old man with close ties with my family and the church, swearing serves only to relieve stress. I do not swear around my grandchildren or children, in most social situations with friends, or in public situations. But swearing in private or at home enables me to relieve pent-up emotions. I am not aware that Marion has ever felt that I was swearing "at" her. For me, and I suspect for many other caregivers, swearing is an emotional safety valve.

However, letting off steam through swearing has limited and only short-term benefit. Swearing reduces my anger, but it does not strengthen positive peace. It merely helps clear away some obstacles to positive peace. As the months of caregiving go by, I can feel the inner pressure slowly increasing. Signs of this building inner pressure are a tightening in my gut and a harder edge to my voice in speaking with Marion. These are indications that my patience is running low, and as my patience and inner peace decline, so does my kindness. Swearing alone does not relieve all my stress, so I rely on another simple practice—physical activity.

### b. Physical activity.

Daily physical activity is a simple way to relieve stress. For me this begins in the morning after I have had breakfast. Every day I do a number of exercises given to me by my physical therapists at various times over the last thirty years. Standing, I begin with twenty repetitions each of four stretch band exercises for my left shoulder. Back in the eighties I tore a rotator cuff tendon in my left shoulder, which has never recovered full strength, but the exercises keep it basically functional. Then I lie down on a mat in our study, and I start out with twenty pelvic tilts and thirty sit-ups. After I catch my breath, I raise a five-pound weight over my head ten times with both arms (that is about all my rotator cuff can take). Then I do twenty repetitions each of four exercises for strength and flexibility in my arms and legs.

Physical activity has always been important to me. Although I was not an outstanding athlete (my high school class had the worst major sport records in our school history), I continued to play my two high school sports—basketball and tennis—as long as I was physically able. Basketball ended for me in my early thirties, and a persistently recurring sore right wrist caused me finally to give up tennis in my early seventies. Since giving up tennis, my main physical activity has been walking. Marion and I are fortunate that we both are able to walk without pain or difficulty. A two-mile walk together in our neighborhood later in the afternoon is our most common practice. But when conditions warrant, we do yard work: Marion trimming bushes, pulling weeds, and raking; I mowing with a push mower, raking, digging in our small garden, or in winter running our small snow blower and shoveling snow here and there. Occasionally in good weather, we do our walk on one of the beautiful trails that border the river running through our town of Decorah.

Marion and I are fortunate in that we do physical activity because we enjoy it and feel refreshed by it. This is not the case for everyone. Yet if caregivers need some extra incentive for being physical active, they should consult the Alzheimer's Association website, which gives these three fundamental "Tips on Being a Healthy Caregiver":

1. See the doctor.
2. Get moving. While thirty minutes of exercise at least five times a week is recommended, even ten minutes a day brings some benefit.
3. Eat well. What is recommended is a Mediterranean diet that has relatively little red meat and emphasizes whole grains, fruits, vegetables, fish, nuts, and olive oil.

For myself, physical activity not only helps release inner tension, but positively it also fosters a meditative awareness of God and kindness toward Marion. Especially when I am walking alone, my mind and heart tend to be drawn toward God and love of Marion. For me walking alone is conducive to my third practice for relieving stress—meditation.

### c. Meditation

The third practice that helps me relieve the stress of long-term caregiving and strengthen patience and kindness is meditation. My usual routine almost every day is to meditate privately for twenty minutes in the morning. I use two traditional forms of Christian meditation that have been nurtured especially in the Eastern Orthodox tradition—*the Jesus Prayer and icons.* After breakfast, I sit in our study with the door closed, and I look straight ahead at a large icon of Jesus. Marion and I have seven icons on the walls of this room, but the largest by far—an icon of Jesus from chest up—has a life-size image of Jesus. While I look directly at this icon, I mentally repeat the Jesus Prayer, "Lord Jesus Christ, have mercy on me."

Raised as a midwestern Lutheran, I had no early life awareness of these practices. I stumbled onto the Jesus Prayer in the late seventies after I had been investigating Transcendental Meditation while writing a denominational Sunday school book on current religious movements. In TM one uses a word (called a mantra) assigned by a TM teacher, repeating the word and letting go of distracting thoughts. Although I found TM to be relaxing, I did not accept its Hindu framework of beliefs. For a while I meditated using the biblical word, *Abba,* the familiar Aramaic word for Father that Jesus used, like the English "Daddy." But after a year or so, I discovered the Jesus Prayer, and I have stayed with it ever since. I usually correlate the prayer with my breath. As I breathe in, I think "Lord Jesus Christ," and as I breathe out I think "Have mercy on me." As I relax more, my breath and the prayer slow down. To be honest, most of the time while I'm meditating with the Jesus Prayer, my mind is going all over the place. I do not let that bother me. I have learned that this is normal. But when I become aware that my attention has drifted, I bring it back to Christ with the words of the Jesus Prayer and the icon before me.

I cannot over-estimate the importance of this meditative practice for my caregiving. *This practice grounds me.* Indeed, the Jesus Prayer comes to me often involuntarily, most frequently when I am alone and walking. I may be simply walking from our car to my office in the Luther College library or walking later from my office to the college coffee shop and that prayer comes to mind. Or during my afternoon walk in our neighborhood, after Marion has left for home, frequently the Jesus Prayer comes to me. At these times, I do not decide, "I'm going to do the Jesus Prayer." It just comes of itself. But this reality is grounded in my regular morning habit of sitting alone in our study praying the Jesus Prayer. So the Jesus Prayer is an incredible comfort for me.

One might wonder how the Jesus Prayer can be such a comfort. If we are accustomed to prayer as talking to God about the concerns of our life and listening for answers to our concerns, then repeating the same few words over and over may seem pointless and boring. However, the great strength of the Jesus Prayer is that it fosters simple awareness of God's presence. For me as Marion's primary caregiver, mindfulness of God's presence is the great stabilizer amid the turbulence of daily responsibilities.

While not everyone will find the particular practice of the Jesus Prayer as their core prayer practice, there are many other possibilities. A considerable variety of meditative prayer practices have developed over the centuries in Christianity. The practice that has been most widely used is some variant of *lectio divina*. This Latin name, which literally means "divine reading," refers to an ancient practice of meditating on a sacred text, usually from the Bible. For instance, one might focus on the opening words of Psalm 23: "The Lord is my shepherd, I shall not want." One might repeat these words several times either out loud or silently, and then let one's attention rest on what stands out; it might be a single word, a phrase, or the whole sentence. Doing *Lectio divina* on the opening words of the twenty-third psalm is not study or rational analysis of those words. Rather, this form of prayer is done with the hope of *experiencing* the Lord *as* one's shepherd, guide, and protector.

The great strength of *lectio divina* is its ability to provide a channel for God to communicate with us in our current situation. What it means for God to be *my* shepherd will differ some from time to time, and it may differ some from what it means for God to be *your* shepherd. Our needs change as our circumstances change. The book of Psalms with its 150 psalms from Israel's worship life more than two thousand years ago is able to provide a meaningful avenue for communicating with God in a great variety of situations. For instance, in the fall of 1994 I had major surgery for colon cancer and endured harsh weekly chemotherapy injections for nearly a year. Very soon after the surgery I read through the whole book of Psalms, but I found special support in Psalm 6, which begins:

> O Lord, do not rebuke me in your anger,
> or discipline me in your wrath.
> Be gracious to me, O Lord.
> for I am languishing;
> O Lord, heal me, for my
> bones are shaking with terror. (Ps 6:1–2)

What especially stood out for me in Psalm 6 were these words in verse 8:

> Depart from me, all you
> workers of evil,
> for the Lord has heard the
> sound of my weeping.

In the days soon after the surgery, I discovered the power of these words in verse 8 for me. Sometimes out loud, sometimes silently, I commanded over and over, "Depart from me, all you workers of evil, for the Lord has heard the sound of my weeping." With these words and God's authority I commanded the colon cancer cells—my "workers of evil"—to leave my body. At first I repeated this prayer from my sick bed, and later as I grew strong enough to take a gradually lengthening daily walk, I repeated those words while I walked in our neighborhood.

One woman, who daily visits her widowed mother with Lewy body dementia in a care facility, has a regular devotional practice of reading Scripture, writing in her journal, and doing a form of meditation called *centering prayer*. In centering prayer we use a single word to direct our awareness toward God. Turning to our own prayer word day after day tends to calm our heart and quiet our thoughts. Of course, our thoughts go this way and that, but when we become aware of this, we gently bring our attention back to our word. As the name suggests, centering prayer helps us find our center in God.

The practice of centering prayer has been advanced since the 1970s especially by two American Cistercian monks, Basil Pennington and Thomas Keating, who advise that one begins with inwardly repeating the chosen word. Naturally, our attention wanders; perhaps by thinking about an event later in the day. When we become aware of this, we return to our word. Soon our attention may turn to a sad memory; again we let go of that sad memory by returning to our word as a way of attending to God's presence. Thomas Keating says:

> We are not attending to a particular thought or object, or even to the sacred word as would be the case in a mantric kind of prayer. Our attention is a general and loving awareness of the presence of God. The actual work of Centering Prayer is consenting to God's presence and in doing so letting go of the present moment with its psychological content. If a thought or feeling stirs unconscious programs along with their commentaries, then before we "get on the boat," we return to the sacred word. With time, patience, and many failures, we develop the habit of letting go of thoughts

promptly—not by thinking about the fact that we are thinking, but simply by returning ever-so-gently to the sacred word.[12]

As Keating says, "The actual work of Centering Prayer is consenting to God's presence." God's presence is an ever-present reality, but most of the time we do not acknowledge that presence. We tend to be preoccupied by memories, feelings, and ideas that make up "the present moment with its psychological content." In Centering Prayer we turn away from that psychological content and recognize the divine presence.

A considerable variety of meditative prayer practices have developed over the centuries in Christian spiritual practice. What is spiritually helpful for one person may not be beneficial for another. So a willingness to try new spiritual practices may lead to a fruitful discovery. Icons have been a fruitful discovery for me.

The word *icon* comes from the Greek word *eikon*, which means image. The ancient Orthodox churches of the Eastern Mediterranean developed the practice of making images of holy persons and sacred events, which are called icons. Icons of Jesus, Mary, and various saints continue to be produced. Those in the Orthodox tradition do not say that an icon is painted; rather, an icon is "written." Traditions of iconography prescribe some particular clothing, color, or object for certain biblical characters. Jesus and the saints all have halos. Jesus wears a red undergarment with a blue outer garment, while Mary's clothing colors are the reverse. Old Testament prophets hold a scroll, while the writers of the four Gospels hold a book. It is abundantly clear that icons are not intended to be photographic. They are visual symbols that invite meditation, and that is how they work for me. When I sit in our study for my morning meditation, my body faced straight ahead to the life-size icon of Jesus, he beckons my heart and mind to focus on him.

Of course, my attention wanders, again and again. But there is always that icon beckoning me to focus on Jesus and his kindness, his patience, his strength. That is the beauty and the power of an icon. It has the stability and centeredness that can and will undergird my life as I continue caregiving Marion.

Indeed, as I write this, I am waking up to the presence of another kind of icon—a living icon that accompanies me every day. This living icon is Marion. She is the saint who has accompanied me for almost sixty years. Like those saints represented in holy icons, she has not been perfect. But as

---

12. Keating, *Intimacy with God* (New York: Crossroad, 1994), 61, 63.

long as I have known her, God has enabled grace to shine in and through her. Now as Alzheimer's disease gradually diminishes her capabilities, that grace continues to shine through in her courage, kindness, patience, and gentleness. Indeed, she has been for me a living embodiment of Paul's virtues.

Although none of the caregivers I interviewed had a devotional practice very similar to mine—centered on the Jesus Prayer or icons—many expressed the importance of their own meditative practices for caregiving. A wife whose husband had Parkinson's disease spoke of the value of reading the New Testament with him. In addition, she said that over the last seven or eight years before his death, she had written numerous stories about events they had shared over the years. When he was in the nursing home, she would read some of her stories out loud in a large public space, so that others besides her husband could hear. She said, "One story—about our falling in love—was called 'Romance Strikes.' At the end of it, everyone applauded. They thought it was a pretty good run at the story. A lot of people find that memories of the past for people, whose memories are failing, are really important."

A non-religious woman caring for her mother said, "I have done some of what I call Oprah meditations that focus on three or four aspects of your life. He talks some, there is soft music in the background. I have all this chatter going on, have all this stuff going on, but I focus on my breathing. It's so difficult, but I do find that I'm more calm afterward. So basically, you're back again and centered—I guess that's the best term for it—centered. So you have a pressure valve."

Another meditative practice that has gained considerable attention is *mindfulness*, a practice rooted in Buddhism. Dr. Cheryl Rezek, a British clinical psychologist, says, "Mindfulness is the process of paying attention to yourself in the context of now."[13] For instance, she suggests taking a walk, slowing one's pace, and then bringing your attention to the sensations of walking.

> Acknowledge any emotions that appear. Take a mental step back from such an active involvement in the environment. Keep your focus on your body and the sensation of moving slowly and with attention. Continue to observe your breathing as a space forms between you and the outside world.[14]

---

13. Rezek, *Mindfulness for Carers* (London: Jessica Kingsley, 2015), 21.
14. Rezek, *Mindfulness for Carers*, 20.

Take a moment to appreciate this moment, knowing you can carry this sense of quietness and clarity with you when you move back into your everyday activities.

Some Christians as well as some non-religious persons use a practice that combines physical movement with meditation—*Tai Chi*. The light, fluid movements of *Tai Chi* have their roots in the worldview of Taoism, the indigenous Chinese religion associated with the Tao Te Ching, a philosophical and political text purportedly written by Lao Tzu sometime in the third or fourth centuries BCE. Many exercise programs such as those at Curves and some physical therapy centers offer *Tai Chi* or something similar. Catholic retreat centers frequently offer group classes on *Tai Chi* and *Tai Chi* videos are readily available.

One might wonder whether it is appropriate for a Christian to use a religious practice rooted in another religious tradition. But the fact is that from time to time throughout history Christians have taken ideas and practices from another faith context and baptized them for Christian use. Many features of Jewish synagogue worship were adapted for Christian worship. The early church fathers in the fourth century used Greek philosophical ideas to affirm the doctrine of the Trinity. The most widely held explanation of December 25 as the date for Jesus' birth is that Christians modified the Roman sun festival on this the shortest day in the Julian calendar. In similar fashion, some Christians today believe it is possible to adapt the Buddhist practice of mindfulness or the Taoist practice of *Tai Chi* for Christian use. Of course, the critical adaptation is to keep awareness of God in Christ as fundamental for the practice.

Distraction is a common difficulty in prayer that we never vanquish in this life. Those who are serious about prayer look for ways to combat distraction and focus more fully on God. One good way to do that is to read and meditate on Scripture. Gazing at a physical symbol is another way. Some find walking or running fosters meditation. For others, the practice of mindfulness or doing some gentle physical movement like *Tai Chi* is an aid in focusing.

### d. Periodic Private Retreat

When I feel my irritability becoming persistent, I turn to a fourth practice: the personal retreat. In order to reduce my irritability and regain a considerable measure of peace, I need to get a significant break from caregiving by taking a full two-day retreat. In some respects, my retreat practice is similar to that of the husband who goes away fishing. Both practices involve going away from home to a quiet place with few or no demands.

For over forty years now I have periodically gone on retreats provided by the community of a Catholic religious order. I started in the mid-seventies at New Melleray Abbey, a monastery of Cistercian monks near Dubuque, Iowa. My first acquaintance with the Cistercians was in reading Thomas Merton, a monk with a Cistercian/Trappist monastery in Kentucky. I still have a special place in my heart for Thomas Merton. Although now I have given away almost all my books, one that I could not give away is Merton's *New Seeds of Contemplation*, which still touches me deeply. Just looking now at this book on a shelf directly in front of me moves my heart with gratitude. Thomas Merton planted seeds in my soul that still produce fruit today.

What have I done on these retreats? It has varied over the years. During about fifteen years of private retreats with the Cistercian monks at New Melleray Abbey, I attended many of the eight "canonical hours" spaced throughout the twenty-four-hour day in which the monks gathered for communal prayer. As a guest, I could not share in their chanting of the psalms, but the Scripture readings and the chanting provided a context conducive to my own reflection and prayer. The break from my own work responsibilities and daily social and family relationships provided me with a fruitful opportunity to reflect on those responsibilities and relationships. Stepping away from my day-by-day life gave me valuable perspective on it. I always gained fresh insight and renewed motivation for my family and work responsibilities.

By the mid-eighties I began doing a periodic private retreat at a community of Franciscan sisters in Dubuque, and since the late nineties I have periodically taken private retreats in one of three hermitages constructed and maintained by the Franciscan sisters of La Crosse, Wisconsin. Each of the three hermitages, located in a village eight miles away from the mother house, is a separate hexagon-shaped little house for one person with its own refrigerator, stove, bathroom, heat, and single bed. The building's three sides toward the access road are built into a hillside. Each of the other three sides has a window facing the woods. Directly in front of the recliner chair is a large picture window. I spend a good portion of my retreat time looking at the woods either from that recliner or from an outside chair on the front porch. When I go on retreat in one of these hermitages, I sleep much more than usual, take a daily long walk in the village, and sit for hours quietly looking at the surrounding woods and reflecting on my life with Marion and the rest of our family. When Marion was in the first stage of Alzheimer's, I felt comfortable leaving her alone during these retreats; but since she moved into the second stage by the summer of 2017, I have had to arrange for one of our children to stay with her. All three of our children have family and work commitments of their own. Our daughter, who lives closest, is almost three hours away, while our two sons are much farther away. So, arranging for one of my retreats requires considerable advance planning.

For instance, several weeks prior to Christmas 2017, I was very tired. My fatigue was increased by my inability to sleep well through the night. I very much wanted to sleep, but after a few hours I would wake up, and stay awake for much if not most of the night. Not surprisingly, I was more often impatient and irritable with Marion. In response to my plea to our three kids for help, our son Carter from Indiana arranged to come to stay with Marion for a few days. On the day he was due to arrive, I left home early and arrived midmorning at the hermitage, located a little more than an hour from home. I soon settled down into a recliner and slept through most of the day and then through the night. I expected to be more alert the following day, but I spent most of that second day also sleeping. After returning home from my retreat, I slept very well through the night and was much more patient and kind with Marion.

Six months later during my next retreat at the same place in early June 2018 our daughter Julie came three hours from St. Paul to stay with Marion for two days. To my surprise, I did not take any naps on my first day of this retreat. I had been sleeping much better over the preceding months, so I was not nearly as fatigued as when I entered the previous retreat. However, on the second day I found myself taking an hour-and-a-half nap in the morning and again in the afternoon. What most amazed me, though, was that throughout my waking hours of this second retreat day the Jesus Prayer coursed through my mind hour after hour. I did not plan it. I did not *decide* to do the prayer other than for my usual morning meditative time. The prayer just came of itself throughout the day and into the evening. What an incredible blessing.

*6. Openness to Unexpected Gifts*

Sometimes grace comes to us in unexpected ways. For instance, one 2018 afternoon when I called Marion from my office to see if she wanted to go with me to the supermarket, she declined because on the spur of the moment her good friend Ag had come for coffee and conversation. When I returned home, Ag had gone, but she had left Marion one of her many Sudoko books with simple numerical puzzles. Marion was buoyed by the visit.

A wife caregiving her husband told of two unexpected experiences of grace:

> One week there were more than the usual bumps in the road, including our cat died. That was a blow. So we were hurting and feeling a little down. It also happened to be Father's Day. We went out for supper. The restaurant was packed even more than usual, so we went into the back room. All the booths were taken, but there was a long table open in the middle of the room. We sat down at one end of the table, and another couple that we didn't know sat at the other end. I thought we would just ignore one another. But the other woman said, "Are you Norwegian?" They were visitors from California, who had been at Vesterheim.[15] We talked for about two hours. She happened to be Italian, and he was a Russian Jew, and I have both Italian and Russian roots. They were just wonderful. We never formally introduced ourselves, but I pieced together enough information and afterward I sent them a note saying how much they had lifted us up. That was a real evening of grace.
>
> And I just appreciate little moments. I think of the young boy at the supermarket who helped me out to the car with the groceries, and he asked, "How has your day been?" And he was so sincere, so solicitous.

I am very fortunate in that Marion and I have a long history of harmony, mutual love, and respect. We are frequently affectionate with each other. My own reality is that I experience this positive harmony here and there in my days, weeks, months, and years of caregiving; nevertheless, this harmony is frequently broken by anger and conflict within me and sometimes with Marion.

It must be very apparent that peace in the positive biblical sense of personal and relational harmony is a goal to aim for, but not a goal easily achieved within the experience of caregiving. Sometimes we as caregivers

---

15. *Vesterheim*, Norwegian for "Western Home," is the National Norwegian-American Museum and Heritage Center, which is located in Decorah.

miss an opportunity to give comfort and peace, and we carry that regret with us. A husband, aided by visits from a hospice nurse, had been caring at home for his beloved wife, who had terminal cancer. She slept alone in their bed, because in her condition it was uncomfortable for her to have him there also. So, for months he slept on the couch in their living room. He said, "One thing—and this is a source of *profound regret*—about two or three nights before she went into hospice at the hospital, I was so wiped out, so tired. She asked me to come lie down with her in bed for a while. I said, 'Not right now, I am so tired.' So I lay down on the couch . . . I am so very sorry that I did that." All of us who do long-term caregiving are liable to miss some opportunities to give comfort.

I find that, in many respects, caregiving is an emotional and spiritual struggle. The struggle is most often within myself, but clashes also happen sometimes between Marion and me. And some caregivers experience conflict with other family members. In this emotional and spiritual struggle, the best we can do is to keep moving toward peace as perfect personal and relational harmony. We are never able to sustain perfect harmony, but I shudder even to speculate on what my life with Marion would be like without the measure of peace that God gives us.

*7. A Major Challenge to Peace is Delusion*

At times our loved one may become upset and speak or act inappropriately, because he or she misinterprets what is going on. For example, an elderly woman saw a threat or offense where there was none. She got very upset when she thought her grandson was fooling around with a young woman other than his wife.

The negative effect of dementia on how a person interprets events came home to me powerfully shortly before Christmas, 2018 as I informed our three adult kids in this email message:

*Brad to Julie, Carter, Kim*

About a week or ten days ago, I was in my college library office around 2 p.m. when my office phone rang and it was Mom.

She said, "Can you come home now?"

I asked, "Is something wrong? Are you OK?"

Again she said, "Can you come home now? I need you to come home."

I said, "OK, I'll be there in just a few minutes."

So I immediately drove home. When I got in the house, I asked her, "What's going on?"

She said, "Are you seeing someone?"

I replied, "Seeing someone! Do you mean a doctor appointment? I saw Dr. Wenner a week ago for my annual physical and everything was fine. You were there with me. So no, I don't have a doctor appointment coming up soon."

She said, "Are you seeing somebody else?"

I said, "You mean seeing some other woman? No! I do not have some other woman on the side. You're my sweetie pie. You're the only woman I'm interested in."

She appeared to relax. After a few more minutes, I returned to my office.

Back at my office, it dawned on me that maybe people with Alzheimer's might have hallucinations. Someone whom I had interviewed about a relative with Parkinson's had mentioned hallucinations occurred with Parkinson's. So I went to the Alzheimer's Association website and asked about hallucinations, and I learned that yes, someone with Alzheimer's or other dementia may have hallucinations. The website defines hallucinations as "false perceptions of objects or events involving the senses." It adds that these occur usually in the later stages of the disease. In my inexpert opinion, Mom has been in the second, middle stage of Alzheimer's for about eighteen months now. Knowing this about Alzheimer's and hallucinations now, I may not be surprised by similar experiences. However, this time it came to me totally unexpected, because I had not been aware of this possibility before.

What prompts me to tell you now is that I think she had another hallucination this morning. As usual I had gotten up first, about 6:30. I shaved, had breakfast, and had just finished brushing my teeth in the bathroom. The door to our bedroom was open and Mom, still in her pajamas, was standing near the door. I said, "Hi, how are you doing?"

She said, "Are you leaving? Going away?"

I said, "I'm just going to my office. This is Monday. Later this week, on Thursday I'm going away for a personal retreat, and Carter and Sophie are coming to stay with you."

She said, "So you're not mad? Not like the guy in my head . . . I guess I was dreaming."

I said, "No, I'm not mad at you. I love you. You're my sweetie pie."

For the last few weeks Mom has taken to watching me leave home every day. Unless she is sleeping late, as I'm leaving in the morning for my office she goes into our study, pulls back the curtain, and watches me back out, and when I wave to her, she waves back as I drive off. Previously she has done this only when I was going out of town for a day or two, but now it has become a daily routine.

I'm very glad that I can be here to support her as she experiences these dreadful changes that Alzheimer's Disease brings. I believe that I can do that well only if I am able to get away every few months for a genuine deep rest. For that I deeply appreciate your help and support. Spelling me for about forty-eight hours enables me to catch up on my rest and return to Mom with a glad, willing heart.

Love,
Dad

On the morning of December 27, 2018, I rose extra early, about 5:45, had breakfast, did my morning exercises, and meditated for almost twenty minutes when Marion came into the study where I was sitting, and said, "I don't want you to go away yet." I told her the college library didn't open for another half hour. She asked me to come to bed with her, so I crawled back into my place in bed and she snuggled up to me. We lay there quietly for several minutes. Then she said, "I want you to know that you're the greatest blessing in life for me." Besides being impressed that she could still articulate such a touching thought, I was profoundly moved by her love. I replied, "You are the greatest blessing in life for me." She said, "Thank you for saying that." She gently touched my face, and I gently touched her face. We lay quietly together for several minutes, and then I got up.

### Peace Within the Family

In addition to peace within the recipient of care and peace within the primary caregiver, the third broad aspect of peace in caregiving is peace within the family. This is the broader social network that in most situations surrounds both the primary caregiver and the recipient of care. It is well to remember that *Shalom*, peace in the biblical sense, is not just an absence of open conflict, but positive harmony and well-being.

As one might expect, the nature of a caregiver's family network is highly variable. Some in-home caregivers have the responsibility entirely on their own. Some caregivers have supportive family members nearby.

## Finding Grace in Caregiving

One woman caring for her husband with Parkinson's had a middle-aged son living a few blocks away, who declared, "I'm ready to come at any time, day or night. I have a sweatshirt by my bed; just call if you need help." Some caregivers have supportive family members who live at a considerable distance, so they appear on scene infrequently.

My daughter and two sons all are willing to help me in caregiving Marion, but their distance from us and their own duties require that we plan ahead. Yet their support and willingness to help are physically and *emotionally* extremely helpful for me. Because of them, I do not feel as though I am alone with this responsibility. Furthermore, their intermittent presence and Facetime conversations help keep Marion connected with them. My situation is similar in this respect to most of those I interviewed, for most felt some measure of support from family members. However, the nature and extent of that support varied greatly.

Among those I interviewed, it was not uncommon to have siblings or one or more children living at a distance of a thousand miles or more. Even if those family members are willing to help with caregiving, ordinarily it has to be planned well in advance. They do not have a sweatshirt by the bed, ready to come when you call for help. When a relative at a distance wants to be involved and to help out, the family member nearby may need to make any major change in care judiciously; when possible, taking time to consult with the distant relative. One man I interviewed noted that one of his challenges has been to make major caregiving decisions jointly with his two siblings who live far away and visit once or twice a year. On occasion when this man has seen the need to make a major caregiving decision, it has taken some effort on his part to give his siblings sufficient time to process the relevant issues, so that they all agree.

In some situations, another close relative may be emotionally as well as physically distant. One woman, who cares for her mother with dementia in a care facility, has just one sibling who lives about six hours away and visits once, maybe twice a year. This caregiver says of her sister, "I think my sister is really very detached from my mom. I think she has already grieved the loss of mom." So, while there may be no open conflict in a caregiver's wider social network, there definitely may not be the positive harmony of *Shalom*.

## Peace as God's Gift

Peace in the caregiving situation is a precious, yet elusive goal for those of us who do caregiving either privately or as our employment. Since the biblical meaning of peace is not merely the absence of fighting, but involves positive harmony and well-being, such peace is a goal toward which to move, but it is not within our power to achieve and maintain. This deeper peace may graciously touch our lives and relationships, yet we are not able to hold on to it. This peace is a gift from God moment by moment. So this deeper peace is not achieved by our direct assault, but is given to us when we open our mind and heart to kindness and love. The Christian faith affirms the eternal reality of such kindness and love in God and proclaims God's overflowing desire to give us that profound peace.

CHAPTER SIX

# Patience

WE WHO ARE LONG-TERM caregivers know that the personal quality we most often find in short supply is patience. And when we are impatient, unkindness is lurking nearby.

Those of us who do caregiving day after day soon discover that patience is difficult to sustain. Indeed, my own search for grace in caregiving began in earnest with the painful awareness that I was short on patience with Marion, and so was unkind to her. The close link between patience and kindness is what first led me to turn to St. Paul for help in caregiving. I recalled that familiar passage in St. Paul's First Letter to the Corinthians where he says, "Love is patient; love is kind." So, in May 2015 I wrote a sermon on those familiar words. In the process of writing that sermon I was reminded that Paul unpacks the nature of love more fully in Galatians 5:22–23, which is the passage from which the reflections of this book flow.

Saint Paul clearly recognized the need for patience in caregiving. Whether one is caregiving fledgling Christian communities around the ancient Mediterranean Sea, as Paul did, or caring for someone with dementia today, patience is greatly needed. So, it is understandable that among the fruit of the Spirit cited by Paul is patience. A biblical understanding of patience has three interconnected aspects.

1. The first aspect of patience is being *slow to anger*. This is a basic quality of God's patience. As Psalm 103:8 says, "The Lord is merciful and gracious, slow to anger and abounding in steadfast love." This Hebrew expression that God is "slow to anger" is often translated in the New Testament with

the Greek word *makrothymos*, the prolonged (*makro*) restraint of anger (*thymos*).

The close link between God's patience and human patience is set forth graphically in Jesus' parable of the Unforgiving Servant (Matt 18:23–35). The parable tells of a slave who owes his king an enormous debt of 10,000 talents (the currency of the day). When the slave cannot pay the debt, the king orders him, his family, and all his possessions to be sold to make the payment. When the slave appeals to the king, "Have patience [*makrothymos*] with me, and I will pay you everything," the king graciously forgives him the entire huge debt. Jesus' parable continues: this slave then encounters another slave who owes him a very small debt. Although this other slave asks him to be patient (*makrothymos*) with him, the first slave refuses and has him thrown into prison. When the master finds out what has happened, he summons the ungrateful slave and says, "Should you not have had mercy on your fellow slave, as I had mercy on you?" Jesus is saying to us that since God is so generous in forgiving our sins, we should be generous in forgiving those who sin against us.

As this parable teaches, being slow to anger is an expression of mercy. Mercy is not present in large areas of our life, because many of our day-to-day social interactions are based on giving and receiving what is due. If we are an employee, we rightly expect to receive the agreed-upon compensation for our work. If we are an employer, we rightly expect quality work from those whom we employ. If we are residents of a city, we expect to receive services such as water, sewer, and garbage pickup as long as we pay for them. Most of social life operates on strict justice, giving and receiving what is due. So, if an employee often fails to show up for work, the employer can rightfully dismiss that employee. If a city resident does not pay what is owed for water and sewer, the water can be turned off. Of course, it is possible for an employer to make special allowance for a worker's difficult circumstances such as serious illness that brings absences beyond what the contract stipulates. That is an act of mercy by the employer. Likewise, a friend of a city resident unable to pay the utility bill may cover that charge; that is an act of mercy. In similar fashion, being slow to anger in caregiving or other human relationships is an expression of mercy.

There is enormous need for being slow to anger in a long-term caregiving relationship. For instance, now one of Marion's frequent early morning behaviors is to dress as though she is going to church. Since she ordinarily gets up considerably later than I do, she is often fully dressed before I notice and tell her it is not Sunday. Of course, this alone is no big deal. But the frequent need to remind her what day it is can be rather trying when I am tired. I thought purchasing an electronic clock that tells day and time would ease the need to remind her about the day of the week, but having its lighted face in our bedroom has not helped. Reminding her what day it is remains a frequent responsibility for me. Fortunately, I have become patient about this and calmly remind her of the day.

Being patient, slow to anger, can be relatively easy for a caregiver when one is well rested and is on good terms with the person receiving care, but being slow to anger is difficult when one is tired or at odds with the recipient of care. I notice in myself that as I get increasingly tired, I get more irritable. For instance, by mid-December 2017 I had been without a thorough rest for about six months. My preconception was that if I was extra tired, I would sleep especially long and well. That turned out not to be the case, for my sleep pattern became disrupted. While I generally fell asleep quickly, I frequently was awake for two or more hours in the middle of the night. Week after week, this took its toll on me. Neither at the time nor in retrospect have I understood why this disrupted sleep kept happening. But the reality was that my cumulative fatigue gradually increased. Not surprisingly, I became more readily irritable, quick to snap at Marion. I could feel my anger close to the surface, ready to erupt. I had to restrain it consciously, but sometimes it broke out anyway.

My greatest test for being slow to anger came on an early December Saturday morning in 2018 as Marion and I prepared to leave home for the supermarket. After putting on my coat and cap, I reached into my pants pocket for my keys and came up with nothing. My key ring with keys to our Honda, our house, and my college mailbox was not there. I looked in vain on the study desk where I usually leave my keys and in a kitchen cabinet where we keep various duplicate keys. Then I searched several of my jackets; still no keys. For a moment I wondered whether I had left my keys in my college office, but I realized that could not be the case, since I had used the Honda key to drive home. I carefully looked around; still no key ring. I became alarmed, because we have only one backup Honda key. I worried what would happen if that too were lost. We have only the one car, and the nearest Honda garage is seventy miles away. I didn't know whether a local locksmith could make a key for the car. I swore vehemently several times, but with great effort sought to contain my frustration and anger. I did not want to attack Marion, although I suspected that she had uncharacteristically taken my keys for some reason. So, I got the backup key from a kitchen cabinet. I hoped that the key ring would resurface. If necessary, we would get another Honda key made one way or another. I calmed down, and we drove to the supermarket.

The next morning after breakfast, by habit I went to pick up my billfold from its usual overnight place on our study room desk. Next to my billfold was my "lost" key ring with the Honda key. I knew I had not put it there. Marion had not said anything to me about the keys, and I did not question her now. Most likely she would not remember the lost key ring from yesterday or how she had found it. Of course, I was glad to have my key ring back, but even more I was glad that I had not attacked her the day before. This also taught me that being slow to anger may not necessarily mean dealing with adversity with complete calm; it may mean just keeping a lid on one's anger for awhile.

A few days later, shortly before Christmas, our son Carter arrived from Indiana to stay two days with Marion while I went away for a private forty-eight-hour retreat. I arrived at the hermitage managed by Franciscan sisters about 10:00 a.m., moved in my luggage and food supplies, and quickly fell asleep in the recliner. I slept about sixteen hours out of the first twenty-four hours there. Although I expected that I would be alert after that, I was surprised to find that I slept much of the second day as well. I had never slept so much in my entire life. When I returned home, I was relaxed and glad to see Marion.

Marion and I are blessed in that we continue to be very close, so we are not dealing with long-held resentments. We hug, kiss, and declare our love for one another often. Not every spousal caregiver has that. One of Marion's memories, recalled from time to time over the years but no longer, was of an event in the last year of her parents' long, rather conflicted marriage. At that late point in their marriage, her father was quite dependent on her mother. He had survived a major heart attack several years before, but he was substantially weakened. They were living then in a small house with two bedrooms, one for her father and one for her mother. One night as they were going to bed, her father with his poor circulation was cold. He asked her mother if he could come into bed with her to get warm, but she refused him. From time to time Marion had recalled this event with great sadness. It is a tragic example that when there is tension and conflict in a relationship, patience is in short supply. Caregiving then becomes especially difficult.

2. The second aspect of the biblical understanding of patience that the apostle Paul and other biblical writers highlight is *calm endurance of difficult circumstances*. The Greek word *kartereo* (from *kratos*, strength) means to remain strong, be steadfast. Paul uses a form of this word when he calls the Roman Christians to "persevere in prayer" (Rom 12:12). This particular message from Paul was timely, for around that time in the city Christians were subjected to periodic harsh persecution by Roman authorities. In similar fashion, a long-term caregiving situation may produce difficult circumstances in which the caregiver feels like quitting, giving up, and walking away. Being patient in caregiving is to hang in there, to continue giving care even through especially trying times.

Extended caregiving presents a multitude of opportunities for patience as calm endurance of difficult circumstances. I walked unaware into one such circumstance one December 2018 weekday afternoon, as I reported in an email to our daughter and two sons.

> Julie, Carter, Kim,
>
> About a week or ten days ago, I was in my college library office around 2 p.m. when my office phone rang and it was Mom.
> She said, "Can you come home now?"
> I asked, "Is something wrong? Are you OK?"
> Again she said, "Can you come home now? I need you to come home."
> I said, "OK, I'll be there in just a few minutes."
> So I immediately drove home. When I got in the house, I asked her, "What's going on?"
> She said, "Are you seeing someone."
> I replied, "Seeing someone! Do you mean a doctor appointment? I saw Dr. Wenner a week ago for my annual physical and everything was fine. You were there with me. So no, I don't have a doctor appointment coming up soon."
> She said, "Are you seeing somebody else?"
> I said, "You mean seeing some other woman? No! I do not have some other woman on the side. You're my sweetie pie. You're the only woman I'm interested in."
> She appeared to relax. After a few more minutes, I returned to my office, puzzled, but not seriously worried.
> At my office, it dawned on me that maybe people with Alzheimer's might have hallucinations. Someone whom I had interviewed about a relative with Parkinson's had mentioned that hallucinations occur with Parkinson's. So I went to the Alzheimer's

Association website and asked about hallucinations, and I learned that yes, someone with Alzheimer's or other dementia may have hallucinations. The website defined hallucinations as "false perceptions of objects or events involving the senses." It added that these occur usually in the later stages of the disease. In my inexpert opinion, Mom has been in the second, middle stage of Alzheimer's for about 18 months now. Knowing this about Alzheimer's and hallucinations now, I may not be surprised by similar experiences. However, this time it came to me totally unexpected, because I had not been aware of this possibility before.

What prompts me to tell you now is that I think she had another hallucination this morning. As usual I had gotten up first, about 6:30. I shaved, had breakfast, and had just finished brushing my teeth in the bathroom. The door to our bedroom was open and Mom, still in her pajamas, was standing near the door. I said, "Hi, how are you doing?

She said, "Are you leaving? Going away?"

I said, "No, I'm just going to my office. This is Monday. Later this week, on Thursday I'm going away for a personal retreat, and Carter and Sophie are coming to stay with you."

She said, "So you're not mad? Not like the guy in my head . . . I guess I was dreaming."

I said, "No, I'm not mad at you. I love you. You're my sweetie pie."

For the last few weeks Mom has taken to watching me leave home. Unless she is sleeping late, as I'm leaving in the morning she goes into our study, pulls back the curtain, and watches me back out, and when I wave to her, she waves back as I drive off. Previously she has done this only when I was going out of town for a day or two, but now it has become a daily routine.

I'm very glad that I can be here to support her as she experiences these dreadful changes that Alzheimer's Disease brings. I believe that I can do that well only if I am able to get away every few months for a genuine deep rest. For that I deeply appreciate your help and support. Spelling me for about 48 hours enables me to catch up on my rest and return to Mom with a glad, willing heart.

Love,
Dad

The next day our daughter Julie, who has a Master of Social Work degree in administration and works for the Minnesota Department of Health, answered me.

> Hi Dad,
>
> Thanks for letting us know about these new developments. I wonder if the idea that you're having an affair is more of a delusion than a hallucination. I also did some reading and found that people with Alzheimer's can have hallucinations (involving seeing, hearing, smelling or feeling things that aren't really there), delusions (false beliefs that the person thinks are real; more than one website gave the example of the person thinking their spouse is in love with someone else), and paranoia (a type of delusion where a person might feel that others are mean, lying, stealing, or "out to get me").
>
> Some tips the websites gave included not arguing with the person; comforting the person if they are afraid; providing reassurance; distracting the person, including moving to another room or going for a walk; not watching violent or fear-provoking shows on TV (it can seem real for that person); having duplicates of things they think are lost or stolen; and avoiding laughing or whispering near the person.
>
> A few of the websites recommended taking the person in to see the doctor if this is new behavior. If you are thinking of doing that and would take her to Mayo, I would be happy to meet you guys there for the appointment.
>
> Thank you for being so loving, caring, and patient with Mom.
>
> Love,
>
> Julie

The various conditions causing dementia call for a caregiver's calm endurance of a variety of difficult circumstances. A very common circumstance is difficulty the person with dementia often has with being alone.

One woman told of the beginnings of caregiving her husband. While visiting family, he had heart pains. Soon he was in the hospital having heart surgery to install stints, but his heart stopped. They had what was called a "code blue." Looking back later, they thought his brain was deprived of oxygen for a time. The wife said, "After that, he sort of hated to have me go anywhere; he didn't like when I wanted to go someplace. For awhile, it would be OK, if I wrote down the phone number of where I was going to be, but then it got so he couldn't use the phone. Then I couldn't be gone. That's when it got harder."

Then I asked my standard question, "What were the major challenges that you experienced in caregiving?" She replied:

> I would say... not having *any* time to myself.... It was like after we would go to bed at night, I would get up and go into the TV room and sit and read for a little while. Then it seemed like two-three minutes, he'd come and say, 'Aren't you coming to bed?' I'd say, 'I'm just going to read a little.' Then in just a few minutes, he'd be asking me, 'Aren't you done now?' I'd say, 'I just want to read a bit more, and then I'll come to bed.' So finally I'd give up and go to bed.
>
> Another thing: he loved to sit in that rocker and look out. I'd come and say, 'I'm going into the bathroom now, and I'm going to take a bath. Is that OK?'
>
> 'Sure.'
>
> I'd hardly be in there a minute, and he'd say, 'Are you OK?' 'Yes, I'm OK.' Then in five minutes he'd be in asking me, 'Aren't you done now?' That sort of thing became for me the most... I have another friend who says the same thing—*just to let your mind go and relax a little.*

I commented, "Another wife I interviewed had a husband with Parkinson's. She would say to him, 'I'm going down stairs to get the laundry,' and before she even got to the bottom of the steps, her husband would call out, 'Where are you?'"

This woman replied, "Being able to *see* you, to actually *see* you, I think. ... I have the laundry in the basement too, and I'd go down there to iron. I'd say, 'Now I'm going down to iron, and I'll be back in a few minutes.' Pretty soon he'd be at the top of the steps calling out. I'd say, 'I'm ironing; I'll be up soon.'"

Caregiving someone with dementia frequently calls for patience as calm endurance of difficult circumstances.

3. The third aspect of patience is perhaps more active, more assertive than being slow to anger and calmly enduring difficult circumstances. *This third aspect is patience as persistence,* continuing to put forth effort. We may say, for example, that it takes patience to learn a foreign language. As adults, we do not learn a foreign language simply by osmosis, and we cannot just sit passively through a language class. We have to strive, we have to work at it. Patience in this case means persistence, staying at a hard task, continuing to work at it. Jesus highlights this active patience in his parable of the widow who persistently presses a bad judge to give her justice.

> In a certain city there was a judge who neither feared God nor had respect for people. In that city there was a widow who kept coming to him and saying, "Grant me justice against my opponent." For a while he refused; but later he said to himself, "Though I have no fear of God and no respect for anyone, yet because this widow keeps bothering me, I will grant her justice, so that she may not wear me out by continually coming." (Luke 18:1–8)

Patience as persistence is not only required when dealing with the one needing care, but also may be required in relating with other family members. An issue mentioned by the son of elderly parents, each with major health problems, was getting his brother and sister, both living far away, on board with major decisions. This required both persistence and waiting for them to agree.

> A challenge has been the perceptions of my brother and sister and their loved ones, at a distance. So that we can all be on the same page, being able to make decisions together. . . . I found that particularly with my brother. He questioned some of the medical recommendations. He wondered whether in "rural Midwest" there would be good medical care. I think we've all had to give one another more time to come to terms with making decisions. That has been a challenge.

Patience is needed in many everyday situations when being with someone at any stage of dementia. For example, during the months when Marion was making the transition from the first stage of Alzheimer's into the second stage, the special cloth for washing my eyeglasses went missing. Every morning before shaving I wash my glasses with soap and water and dry them with a soft cloth. For over a decade I had used a cloth that was ideal for that purpose—an old cloth baby diaper that was 100 percent cotton and was both very soft and absorbent. Pure cotton cloth is rare today, for if the fabrics used in garments have any cotton, the cotton is generally combined with a synthetic fiber that is not absorbent. Since the diaper was rather large, I kept it under our bathroom counter in a fairly wide and deep drawer that also contained some of Marion's personal items. One day after Marion had done the weekly wash, the diaper was missing. I looked in a kitchen drawer that has the washcloths and towels that we routinely use for washing and drying dishes. There was the baby diaper. I returned it to the usual bathroom drawer, and reminded Marion that I like to have the cloth in that place. Several weeks later, though, the old diaper disappeared again on wash day. But it was not in the kitchen where I had found it before, and not in any other place I checked. It was almost two years later that the diaper mysteriously reappeared. Naturally, I did not bother to ask her where she found it, because she would not remember anyway. Now I keep the diaper in a different bathroom drawer that she does not ordinarily open.

Looking for misplaced household items is not uncommon when living with someone with dementia. When Marion and I are in the kitchen preparing supper, she will frequently look in several places for a utensil and then ask me about it. When I reflect on this, I am amazed at how much information about kitchen items our memory is called upon to store. For instance, the twenty-four-inch-wide top drawer just to the left of our stove contains thirty-seven utensils, several of them variations of the same kind of utensil. Right below the overhead cabinet with large flour and sugar containers is an eighteen-inch wide drawer that has a mixture of various measuring cups and spoons, an assortment of other kitchen utensils, as well as two screwdrivers and a pair of pliers; thirty-seven items in all. These two drawers have the most numerous kitchen items, but the total number of things stored in our kitchen cabinets is considerably larger still. In addition, two sliding doors open to a pantry that has cans and packages of various food items on four shelves as well as on the floor. Since Marion often does not remember where items go, utensils tend to migrate here and there. So as a husband taking over primary responsibility for food preparation, I often have to search for the utensil I want, or settle for an available substitute. Fortunately, after several years, for the most part, I have learned to make do with what I can find at the time. Oh, sometimes when frustrated about not locating the utensil I want, I'll break out with a swear word, but I do not attack Marion personally.

I have found that the best way to monitor my own caregiving is to check frequently the level of my personal patience. Patience is not static. My patience rises and falls as circumstances change, and my readiness to deal with those circumstances in a kind way fluctuates. It would be great to have a patience thermostat on my body like the thermostat in our home that measures temperature and adjusts the furnace or air conditioning to keep our dwelling's temperature at a steady comfortable level. A body-mounted patience thermostat would measure my patience level and regulate it by automatically adjusting my emotional cooler or heater when needed. A patience thermostat would keep me in a comfortable range with only slight variations. Joy, peace, kindness, generosity, and gentleness would come far more readily. But since I lack a patience thermostat, I have to be attentive to my level of patience and make conscious adjustments.

The most common indication that my patience has declined below the desired level is my irritability. The first outward sign of irritability in me is a hard edge to my voice. Next is uttering an expletive. The indication that my patience has fallen further into the danger zone is when I have an angry outburst that lasts longer than one or two expletives. Below that yet is what two wives, who were the primary caregiver for their husbands with dementia, called their "meltdown." By that one woman meant "totally fall apart, break down, be at your wit's end." Since we are human without a mechanical patience thermostat, it is important for us to monitor our own level of patience and, if possible, make appropriate adjustments before reaching a meltdown. I've been fortunate so far in that I have not reached a meltdown.

What can we do to avoid an angry outburst or a meltdown? Some relief from caregiving with genuine rest is needed. A good night's sleep or a good nap is temporary relief from caregiving; both are beneficial for sustained caregiving. But if we become seriously sleep deprived, we need more rest than that. My interviews with home caregivers and my own experience reveal two things as most helpful.

One is to bring in some part-time help from either a professional person or family member. Several people I interviewed spoke very positively of acquiring professional help. A wife caring at home for her husband with Parkinson's, said, "We had . . . home care twice a week, while he was at home. They bathed him, dressed him; they would change the bed, do the laundry, and light housekeeping. That was great support." Even after her husband entered a nursing home this woman continued to have professional home care, "not twice a week, but twice a month. That was very helpful for me. I'm getting older too; I'll be seventy-nine next month."

Another wife of a husband with Parkinson's said:

> And I got [paid] help in, and that was good. I had to have time to do my own business, my own doctor appointments, and such. And I couldn't really leave him alone. I had to go do errands. . . . That's when I got help in, to help him get out of bed in the morning, showered, get breakfast, ready for going down for his nap again. . . . I don't remember how long we had them. I had them for several years anyway.

Although not everyone can afford to pay for professional home health care, it is a very good option for those who can.

Certain long-term care insurance policies provide some reimbursement for home health care after a waiting period. Medicare pays for some home health care services, but not for homemaking assistance. Medicaid and Medicare cooperate in Programs of All-Inclusive Care for the Elderly (PACE), which offer limited health care assistance in thirty-two states.

In some situations, regular relief from full-time caregiving may come from a nearby willing family member. Indeed, in some cases, if possible, it is especially prudent for an elderly individual or couple to move close to a family member who is supportive. As one middle-aged daughter commented about her parents, "When Mom and Dad moved up here by me, they moved away from being by my sister. One part of that was that my community has excellent resources and my sister's community does not. The other part of that was that my dad felt I was better equipped emotionally to handle the next part of the journey for them, that he saw coming. My sister's emotions often override the welfare of others."

As one especially supportive daughter of her mother with Lewy body dementia noted,

> Early on, when Mom and Dad lived at a distance from me, my support was to call them once a week, make sure Dad was OK, and send them mail. They both were really pleased to get mail.
>
> Then when they moved by me four years ago, a fifteen-minute drive away, it was reasonable for me to see them every day. Dad was still strong and able to take care of most of her needs. I'd help with her hair and shopping for clothes, and actually baby sit with her while Dad went out and had some time without worrying, "Is Mom OK now?" That was our routine for the three-and-a-half years before she moved into the care facility. Then when she moved to the care facility, Dad and I would tag team seeing her. At first, if Dad saw her during the first three months, she expected to go home with him. So during those first three months in particular, I was the constant presence with her, and Dad went a couple times a week at most. And that was good for him. He slept a lot and even went fishing.

Another very important factor that affects our patience as a caregiver is a positive relationship with the recipient of care. While patience fosters kindness, it is also true that kindness fosters patience. We are much more likely to be patient with a person toward whom we have a positive, kindly disposition. The long-term coolness in the marriage of Marion's mother and father led her elderly mother to refuse him the temporary warmth and comfort of her bed for his chilled body. An active history of resentment toward the person needing comfort breeds conflict and unkindness. Whenever there is tension and conflict in a relationship, patience is likely to be in short supply and caregiving becomes especially difficult.

The three aspects of patience—being slow to anger, calmly enduring difficult circumstances, and persistence—are not totally different like a stone, a cloud, and cat; that is, clearly different realities. Rather, the three aspects of patience—being slow to anger, calmly enduring difficult circumstances, and persistence—are three aspects of the one complex reality of patience. All of us who do caregiving, whether as professionals or in our family, have great need for patience.

CHAPTER SEVEN

# Kindness

KINDNESS IS FUNDAMENTAL TO all constructive, positive human relationships and interactions, whether in the family, in relations among friends, in business transactions, or wider community relations. However, kindness is especially important in caregiving, because the person receiving care is particularly vulnerable. Since recipients of care may not be able to assert their claim to good treatment, they depend on the goodness, the kindness of their caregiver.

The classical Greek adjective for "kind"—*xrastos*—had the basic meaning of "good," and was applied to things as well as people. A thing is good, *xrastos*, if it fulfills its function well. So one could speak of a good (*xrastos*) coat or a good (*xrastos*) pair of shoes. This usage appears in Jesus' parable about wine at a marriage feast (Luke 5:33–39). Jesus says, "And no one puts new wine into old wineskins; otherwise the new wine will burst the skins and will be spilled, and the skins will be destroyed. But new wine must be put into fresh wineskins. And no one after drinking old wine desires new wine, but says, 'The old is good [*xrastos*]'"

Similarly, a person could be described as good in regard to a certain ability or function. So, someone could be said to be a good (*xrastos*) cook or a good (*xrastos*) farmer. This basic sense of goodness in the sense of serviceability, of fulfilling a function well, was also applied to persons *as they related to other persons*. So in classical Greek literature a man who was good in relation to other people was said to be *xrastos*—helpful, friendly, kind.

# Finding Grace in Caregiving

1. *Being kind involves two basic personal movements: perceiving a need and trying to meet that need. Both movements are required.*

It is possible to not perceive a need through ignorance, general hard-heartedness, or ill will toward the specific person or group. It is also possible to perceive a need in an animal, individual person, or group, yet ignore the animal, individual person, or group in need. Even worse, one might try to take advantage of that need. Some people are hard-hearted; they recognize the need, yet do nothing to help. Other people are like vultures that have a sharp eye for the needs of others and then swoop in to take advantage of it. Those who are kind perceive the need and try to meet that need.

While in the abstract being kind may seem easy, in actual life situations often it is more difficult to carry out. For instance, Marion and I had seven members of our family for Thursday 2018 Thanksgiving dinner at our house, and four of them stayed over two or more nights. After everyone had left on Saturday, Marion did laundry and I cleaned the lower floor bathroom used by our overnight guests. Sunday afternoon I did some vacuuming of our entry way and living room, and Marion was preparing to vacuum the stairs to the lower floor with a canister vacuum cleaner. However, we have two canister vacuums by different manufacturers, each vacuum with its own set of implements, which were mixed up together in a box. For vacuuming the steps Marion wanted to use a small upholstery tool on the end of the vacuum hose, but she could not find a tool that would fit. I offered to help, but she rebuffed me. Feeling miffed, I huffed off to clean the main floor bathroom. After a few minutes, though, my heart softened, and I returned and found the implement that fit on her vacuum hose. She thanked me, and each of us continued with our tasks. While the next day most likely she had no memory of this interaction, I remembered it and felt ashamed of my initial hard-hearted impatience. What this incident taught me, though, is that often my doorway to kindness toward Marion is a period of stepping away from her, even just for a few minutes. Let my irritation subside and my good will increase.

I am extremely fortunate in that Marion has such a kind heart, and I am the primary beneficiary of her kindness. Even when I have been short-tempered or huffy with her, she does not hold it against me. So later on the night of this vacuuming incident, Marion had gone to bed a few minutes before me. When I joined her, she rolled over to me and kindly whispered, "I'm awful glad you're my husband."

## Kindness

I replied, "I'm very glad you're my wife."

She said, "*Mange tusen takk.*" [Norwegian for "many thousand thanks."]

I said, "*Mange tusen takk.*"

"I love you."

"I love you."

However, even though Marion is herself such a kind person, sometimes I find it difficult to be kind to her. To be fair, though, I think I have made progress in adapting to Marion's memory loss. To a considerable extent I now take her lack of memory for granted. As I reflect back on my several years of gradually increasing care for Marion, I see that now without getting angry I routinely accept some things she does that used to irritate me. This dawned on me a few days ago as I searched through several kitchen drawers and cabinets for a particular measuring cup. When the cup was not in its customary place, I automatically looked into several other places. Whereas a year or two ago, this would have elicited a few angry words from me; now I searched calmly until I found it. Searching for kitchen items has become normalized.

By late June 2019 I had made further progress in normalization. One evening after Marion had done our weekly clothes washing, I could not find my summer pajamas. I checked likely drawers and closets, but could not find my pajamas. Even after a broader search, no pajamas. So, I calmly put on a t-shirt and boxer shorts, and they have served me well. I suspect someday my summer pajamas will surface, but I have discovered they are not essential.

My guess is that many of us in caregiving gradually adjust to behaviors that initially annoyed us. For example, following one of the first times our daughter Julie spent two full days with Marion while I went off on retreat, Julie commented in her email report, "I think Mom and Dad must often have potatoes for dinner because it really seemed to confuse her when I didn't want one. She must have asked me twenty times within about seven minutes if I wanted a potato." Although it seems unlikely that Marion literally asked her twenty times, it *felt* like that to Julie. As I think back to my own experience of watching my father calmly tell and retell Mom what day it was, I think answering her about this had become normalized for him. Where there is an underlying kindness toward the person with a memory deficit, we are likely to adjust calmly to behavior that at first annoyed us.

A good number of other "new" behaviors have become normalized for me over the last several years. For instance, it used to be that Marion was directly informed by email or phone about who was hosting her Thursday afternoon Menders coffee group, and Marion would drive herself to and from the gathering. But Marion ceased using email several years ago, then she stopped driving, and now she readily gets confused about a phone message. So the current routine is that I receive an advance email from a neighborhood Mender who tells us both where the group will meet and who will give Marion a ride. A similar change has occurred prior to her monthly gathering of the contemplative Mary circle. Members of both groups take care of her.

I have discovered, though, that while some formerly irritating behaviors may become normalized, the person with dementia is very likely to adopt some fresh behaviors that annoy. I discovered this a few weeks prior to Christmas 2018. One daily routine that Marion and I share is to have tea together sometime mid-afternoon. Marion and I became attached to drinking tea when we spent a year in England directing a Luther College study abroad program in the mid-1970s. We learned to put boiling water into the cup or teapot that has tea and let the tea steep for a few minutes. That has been our customary practice ever since. However, by late 2018 Marion had lost the ability to tell when the water in our tea kettle is boiling. The reliable indication is that our tea kettle whistles when the water comes to a boil. Now apparently Marion thinks the water is ready when it produces the soft rumbling sound of water becoming hot a couple minutes prior to boiling. The result is that the tea is weak and sometimes barely more than lukewarm. Several times I protested about the tea and asked again that the water boil. But after a few weeks of frustration over this, I gave up. After all, in the grand scheme of things, lukewarm tea is not a great hardship. So, I have adapted. Either I handle our afternoon tea making myself or if she does it, I drink weak lukewarm tea without complaint.

Kindly caregiving is not only helped by normalization of accommodating behavior, but also by being sensitive to how much dementia increasingly requires a person to give up. The fundamental movement in an act of kindness is to recognize a need. Being kind to someone with dementia involves some sensitivity to what dementia does to a person: by gradually losing comprehension of language, persons with dementia gradually lose understanding of their physical and social environment.

*2. Loss of language is especially critical*

Language gives us some comprehension of our environment, and thereby *language gives us some measure of appropriate response to and control over our social and natural environment*. For instance, in our *social* environment, as an infant if I link the word *Mama* with the person who cuddles and feeds me, I will welcome the announcement of Mama's presence and look to her for safety, whereas I will be hesitant with a stranger. As an elderly parent, if I know that "Julie" is my daughter, I will smile when Julie comes into view. Understanding certain words also helps us also avoid dangers in wider society. For example, while at an evening program of a large Korean church in Los Angeles in the summer of 2018, I commented to our California son that I intended to walk about a block to a nearby McDonald's for a chocolate shake. He warned me that would be unsafe to do in that neighborhood.

Language also gives us some understanding and control of objects and forces in our *natural* environment. If I understand that "teapot" refers to the metal container for heating water on top of our stove, I can respond appropriately to a request for tea. If I understand the words *thunderstorm* and *lightning*, and the close link between them, I will avoid taking a shower or bath when I'm informed that a thunderstorm is near. If I understand that "lyme disease" is transmitted by "mosquitos," I am more likely to apply insect spray when I mow the lawn. In simple and complex ways, with language we are able to steer through our world with some appropriateness and safety. Language gives us some measure of control over both our natural and social environment.

Recognizing this function of language increases understanding of what it may be like for those who are losing more and more of their language comprehension. If I am losing my memory, someone whom I formerly recognized and valued as a friend, I may now perceive as a stranger, maybe even a threat. At some point I may not recognize formerly beloved family members.

As I lose more and more comprehension of language, a natural and social world that I previously navigated with confidence now becomes a strange, at times threatening environment. It may be like trying to find our way around a strange foreign city where we do not know anyone and do not speak the local language. The uncertainty and feeling of being at risk make us feel vulnerable. This loss of control may be what it is like sometimes for the person with dementia. Recognizing this function of language may help us understand and empathize with the sometime fearful and hostile reactions of our loved one with dementia. Recognizing a need is the first step toward kindness.

Experience shows that dementia does not happen evenly in all parts of our brain. Music is especially resilient for many. I saw this in Flo, who had given piano lessons to many kids in her home. The day I visited her in a local memory care unit, she was not able to talk much, but then she went to the piano in the common room of that unit and with a broad smile on her face began to play and sing.

In another community, a woman in a care facility with advanced Alzheimer's was upset and troubled when her son arrived. He said:

> The other evening she assaulted her roommate and she was very agitated, and the staff had come in and everyone was separated. I just came in and started singing. She has a deep reservoir of hymns. I have found that one of the places Alzheimer's hasn't invaded is that repertoire of hymns. I just kept pulling out a different memorized hymn. There was no order to it (laugh), just that, "She knows this one." I have just seen the power of that on her, on her emotional and spiritual level, and it's something we share together. So I've found that practice has given me the opportunity to connect with her still, when most of the time we are very distant, because of her memory loss.

Nancy Darling, Oberlin College Professor of Psychology, cites a study in which Alzheimer's patients in a nursing home were observed with or without music.

> When listening to music, patients were less agitated, seemed less uncomfortable (engaging in repetitive behaviors indicating nervousness), less vocal, and seemed more positive and calm. In this case, all patients listened to the same music. Even with no special associations with the music other than that it was familiar music they had heard when they were younger (Beatles), positive effects were found.[1]

While general familiarity with the music tends to have a positive effect, Professor Darling says that most people have a stronger and more positive response to music that they knew and liked during their teen years.

---

1. Darling, "Music and Dementia: It Won't Cure Dementia, but It's a Simple Intervention That Will Help." *Psychology Today*, May 5, 2013, https://www.psychologytoday.com/us/blog/thinking-about-kids/201305/music-and-dementia.

It might be popular, classical, opera, or religious music. Those with hearing loss may benefit from headphones. It is important to note that familiar music can do more than keep someone quiet and happy; it may also make deep emotional connections. Professor Darling comments, "My father died two weeks ago. The very last thing he responded to was music as his pastor and my mother sang hymns for him and I accompanied them on recorder. His eyes opened and he reached out and squeezed the pastor's hand. That was a gift indeed."[2]

Kindly caregiving is not only helped by normalization of accommodating behavior, but also by being perceptive to how much dementia increasingly requires a person to give up. I know that reminding myself of how much Marion has already given up helps me be more sensitive to her needs. For instance, over the last several years I have seen Marion gradually decline in her capability to understand and to converse about what is happening around her and within her. Most obvious is her inability to come up with the proper word for an object, activity, or feeling. To be sure, all of us, including the young, experience this memory gap now and then, and to fill the gap we may speak of a "whatcha-ma-call-it." For quite a few years now, Marion's favorite go-to word for this had been "thing-a-ma-jigger." She has ceased to use that term and has resorted simply to "thing." As she searches in our coat closet, she may say, "I'm looking for my thing." Naturally, that does not help me much in understanding what specifically she is looking for. But even more, it must be frustrating for her to be trapped within a world that she is less and less able to understand and talk about with others.

Language is not only our most developed way of communicating with others; it is also our own fundamental way of understanding the world and events that are happening around us. For instance, on a summer day I hear a very loud sound coming from above, and someone nearby says, "It's thunder." If I understand some basic information about thunder, that it is linked with lightning and often accompanies a rainstorm, then I can take appropriate action to find safety from the threat. If I hear my spouse say, "I love you," and I understand those simple words and recognize my spouse, the words comfort me. Language is the basic means by which we orient ourselves to our physical and social environment. As our understanding of language diminishes, our ability to respond appropriately to people and events diminishes. Our environment feels more and more alien.

---

2. Darling, "Music and Dementia," para. 12.

Indeed, one day Marion and I were having our customary afternoon tea in our living room; as usual each of us had pulled a chair to where we sit side by side looking directly out into the woods behind our house. After a few minutes Marion pointed at something outside that she wanted to call to my attention, but she could not come up with the appropriate words to tell me what it was. I made several guesses, but each time she shook her head. After a silent pause, she gave up. Sadness was written on her face. Seeing this very bright, articulate woman so reduced also made me sad.

I suspect that it is even more trying for Marion consistently not to know the names of the people with whom she interacts regularly. When I'm informed by email of where her Thursday afternoon Menders group is meeting each week, I tell her and I also leave a note with the information by our kitchen telephone. Frequently the name of the host person is not enough to help her understand who she is, and I generally offer some description of the host and where she lives. Sometimes this helps; other times it does not. Marion operates not only within an increasingly unintelligible physical world, but also an increasingly unintelligible social world.

Even the innermost portions of her social world are becoming less and less understood by her. For example, soon after the 2018 Thanksgiving visit of our three kids and two of our grandchildren, I happened to reflect on what memories are already shaky or lost for Marion. It has been evident for more than a year that she is shaky about the names and basic biographies of our children, grandchildren, and in-laws. So prior to the arrival of family for Thanksgiving, several times I had reminded her about them. On a several occasions, I said, "Our son Kim and his boy Bryce are coming first from California and will arrive here the Sunday before Thanksgiving." Then closer to Thanksgiving, I told her two or three times that our daughter Julie and her husband Monchy are coming from St. Paul the evening before Thanksgiving. I also told her that our son Carter and his daughter Elsa were coming from Valparaiso, Indiana the evening before Thanksgiving; Carter's wife Michelle would be working and wouldn't be coming. Carter and Elsa would stay with Mary Jane, Michelle's mom. They would all join us for Thanksgiving dinner on Thursday.

Just think how much information is packed into those few sentences! And this information is not about tangential matters, but about those persons who are nearest and dearest to us. Consider what it must feel like to be shaky in one's awareness of these dear, dear people. So it touched my heart to have Marion ask me the morning after Thanksgiving, "Who is the man staying with the boy?" I responded, "That is our son, Kim, and the boy is his son, Bryce. They have come from California."

It must be awful for Marion to navigate a world of which her understanding is so shadowy. Thus far, Marion has always been aware of who I am. But at some point, that memory also will become shaky and eventually lost. In the meantime, it is a precious gift to have her snuggle up to me at bedtime and say that she loves me. To assure her of my love and support for her is my highest purpose in life. Could there be any greater inducement toward kind treatment of her?

## 3. Jesus' Teaching on Kindness

In two of his parables Jesus has much to teach us about the nature and scope of kindness.

The more familiar parable is of the Good Samaritan in Luke 10:25–37:

> Just then a lawyer stood up to test Jesus. "Teacher," he said, "what must I do to inherit eternal life?" He said to him, "What is written in the law? What do you read there?" He answered, "You shall love the Lord your God with all your heart, and with all your soul, and with all your strength, and with all your mind; and your neighbor as yourself." And he said to him, "You have given the right answer; do this, and you will live."
>
> But wanting to justify himself, he asked Jesus, "And who is my neighbor?" Jesus replied, "A man was going down from Jerusalem to Jericho, and fell into the hands of robbers, who stripped him, beat him, and went away, leaving him half dead. Now by chance a priest was going down that road; and when he saw him, he passed by on the other side. So likewise a Levite, when he came to the place and saw him, passed by on the other side. But a Samaritan while traveling came near him; and when he saw him, he was moved with pity. He went to him and bandaged his wounds, having poured oil and wine on them. Then he put him on his own animal, brought him to an inn, and took care of him. The next day he took out two denarii, gave them to the innkeeper, and said, 'Take care of him; and when I come back, I will repay you whatever more you spend.' Which of these three, do you think, was a neighbor to the man who fell into the hands of the robbers?" He said, "The one who showed him mercy." Jesus said to him, "Go and do likewise."

Both the priest and Levite see the obvious need of the assaulted man, yet neither makes an effort to meet that need. They fail to be kind. It is the Samaritan who both sees the great needs of the injured Jew and takes care to provide for those needs. He administers basic first aid by pouring oil and wine on the man's wounds to clean them and provide an antiseptic. Then the Samaritan puts the injured Jew on his own animal and takes him to an inn, where he continues to take care of him. The next day before departing the Samaritan pays the innkeeper to care for the injured man until he returns.

The crucial difference of the Samaritan from the priest and Levite is that the Samaritan "was moved with pity" for the injured man. There was an emotional connection established, the emotion of compassion. New Testament scholar Francois Bovon says of the Samaritan, "Unlike his two predecessors, he let himself be moved. . . . He was moved with compassion. A relationship was established between the wounded man and the Samaritan."[3] The Greek verb that Luke uses here—translated as "moved with pity"—literally means to be moved in one's gut, one's intestines, and it is this same word that Luke uses elsewhere to speak of the compassionate love of God and of Christ.[4] While kindness is rooted in compassion, it bears fruit with helpful action. The Samaritan administered first aid to the injured man, took him to an inn and cared for him, and the next day paid the innkeeper to continue providing care.

Luke underscores this message with the teaching of Jesus in Luke 6:27–35, in which Jesus says to love even our enemies.

> But I say to you that listen, Love your enemies, do good to those who hate you, bless those who curse you, pray for those who abuse you. If anyone strikes you on the cheek, offer the other also; and from anyone who takes away your coat do not withhold even your shirt. Give to everyone who begs from you; and if anyone takes away your goods, do not ask for them again. Do to others as you would have them do to you.
>
> If you love those who love you, what credit is that to you? For even sinners love those who love sthem. If you do good to those who do good to you, what credit is that to you? For even sinners do the same. If you lend to those from whom you hope to receive, what credit is that to you. Even sinners lend to sinners, to receive

---

3. Bovon, *Luke 2: A Commentary on the Gospel of Luke 9:51—19:27* (Minneapolis: Fortress, 2013), 58.

4. Bovon, *Luke 2*, 58.

## Kindness

as much again. But love your enemies, do good, and lend, expecting nothing in return. Your reward will be great, and you will be children of the Most High; for he is kind to the ungrateful and the wicked. Be merciful, just as your Father is merciful.

*The issue is not so much whether we are ever kind, but to whom we are kind. It is helpful to distinguish three circles of possible recipients of our kindness.*

### 1. Being kind to those who are kind to us

The smallest circle includes only those who are kind to us. This is not to be ignored or thought morally insignificant, for this circle likely includes those who love us and those whom we love in return. These are our most dear relationships and with these people likely occur the instances of kindness that are most emotionally meaningful for us. What comes to mind first for me is my dad's sustained kindness toward my mother in their later years when her memory was failing from small strokes. During this period they lived with Marion and me for fifteen months, and day after day I heard Dad respond calmly to Mom's oft repeated question, "What day is it today?" To be sure, Mom and Dad were very close with one another, yet having to repeat oneself again and again can be so trying that an angry response is not unreasonable. Yet Dad was kind to this woman who, fifty years earlier, had been kind enough to stay with him through his years of alcoholism.

During the 2018 Thanksgiving time visit of our three children and two of our grandchildren, there were many instances of kindness. Two stand out in my memory. One was our grandson Bryce's kindness toward Marion during his stay with us. I counted five times when she asked him, "How old are you now?" Every time Bryce answered without a trace of irritation, "I'm eleven." Our son Kim also showed kindness one afternoon as he sat with Marion and me in our living room. Marion began to relate a recurring event from the early weeks after Kim joined our family at age four-and-a-half. She recalled a fragment of a memory. She said to him, "You had your legs around me," but she could not say more. Without a hint of reproach, he quietly added, "You were cooking, and you had me around your waist. I was holding on to you." What a precious memory for both of them. At some point Marion's memory of that interaction will be lost to her. Indeed, just a few minutes earlier, shortly before Kim joined us in our living room, Marion asked me, "Who is that with the boy?" I answered, "That is our son, Kim. His son is Bryce." She will lose her memory of those treasured moments with the child Kim, but those moments will remain a cherished memory for Kim.

For all of us, it is likely that this inner circle of relationships is where we live the most significant portion of our life. Here we are most likely to be kind to those who are kind to us.

*2. Being kind to those we respect*

A wider circle of relationships embraces those individuals that we respect. Of course, we may respect those who belong in our innermost circle, but we respect many other people as well. To respect someone is to have some degree of appreciation and esteem for that person. We may not agree with all that person's beliefs, values, and actions, yet our respect conveys a measure of esteem for that person. So the person who holds those beliefs and values and carries out those actions is regarded as worthy. We give respect to those who in some way measure up to one or more of our value standards. For example, in contemporary America there are widely contrasting views about gun ownership. It is possible for members of the same family to have significant disagreements on this issue, yet have respect for one another. A non-gun owner may respect a sibling who loves to hunt pheasants and carefully locks up the gun between hunts. In turn the hunter may show respect for the non-hunter's convictions about guns in American culture, while disagreeing with those convictions.

In similar fashion, I have some relatives and friends with whom I have deep differences on politics, yet we show respect for one another and are kind toward one another. When I meet these relatives, we hug and express genuine affection, and we do the same when we part. While we are together, ordinarily we refrain from verbal barbs that we might use with strangers or opponents. Here respect is joined with brotherly/sisterly love. Some of my friends share my views on topics on which many people deeply divide—politics and religion—but I also have some friends with whom I have deep differences on these topics. In spite of our differences, though, we tend to avoid sharp conflict, and we manifest kindness toward one another by expressing concern and support when difficulties arise.

A bit further out within this second circle are some acquaintances whom we respect. An acquaintance is someone we recognize and greet politely, but do not know well. For example, I am acquainted with Marion's primary care physician. I go with Marion when she has a medical appointment with this person, who, it just so happens, often sits a row or two ahead of Marion and me at church on Sunday mornings. If one day this woman came to church with her right arm in a sling, without hesitation I would offer to help with her two young children's coats. She is a respected acquaintance that I am predisposed to trust and help.

Yet a little further out in this second circle are persons we do not know personally, yet they belong to a group that we generally trust and respect. For example, if I received a communication from Pastor Arote Vellah in Zimbabwe that a colleague of his was coming to my town, I would gladly offer to host and assist that person even though I have never met the person. The key is that the visitor comes with a recommendation from a person I trust. My personal connections with Arote Vellah go back to the early 1980s, and because Arote Vellah vouches for this visitor, I will welcome the person.

Even further out in this second circle are some public figures that we respect. For me two such public figures are Massachusetts Democratic Senator Elizabeth Warren and Republican former President George W. Bush. I have never met either of them, yet I appreciate their service to our country.

Since in one way or another we respect people in this second circle, we are inclined to be kind toward them.

3. *Being kind to those we dislike, distrust, or fear*

The people in this third circle are those for whom we have negative feelings that range from mild dislike through distrust to full-blown fear. With those we dislike, we try to minimize our involvement by avoiding them as much as possible. With those we distrust or fear, we try to keep our distance, and if they come near, we have our guard up.

Jesus' parable of the Good Samaritan puts the focus on the social relationship between a person's "in" group and those from an "out" group. Although Jews and Samaritans historically had common social and religious roots in ancient Israel, in Jesus' time they had been divided for several centuries. Samaritans and Jews were suspicious and hostile toward one another. Jews tended to look down on Samaritans. We too distinguish between individuals that we like and do not like and between groups that we tend to trust and distrust. The strong emotions elicited powerfully exhibit a contemporary form of the ancient Jew-Samaritan division.

This division between those we like and those we dislike may also play out in caregiving situations. Some senior residents in care facilities are largely ignored by members of their family. Of course, it is very possible that the person has not been good to his or her family. So they may have cause to dislike that person. Nevertheless, Jesus calls us to be kind even to those we dislike, distrust, or fear.

I mentioned this issue to a CNA (Certified Nursing Assistant). "One of the things I hear about nursing homes is that some residents get visits from family members and others who do not."

The CNA replied:

> Yes, absolutely. There are some families—the relatives don't even live here, but they fly here and bring gifts to the resident here. But it's sad to see other residents who have family in the next town, and they never visit.
>
> Some who come to the nursing home think they will get better and go home. But they don't. Then their light just turns off. Their light just becomes dark. That's when we get closer there. They are lonely. We see they need not just a worker, but someone to be closer with them.
>
> One man there said my name was Angel. I don't really talk about that with people or my co-workers. One co-worker said, "He talks about Angel did this or Angel did that." I didn't say anything. This guy is blind, but he recognizes your voice and your smell. Every person has a smell. One day I went to work, and he was screaming and yelling. So I went in and took his hand and talked to him softly. "How are you doing?"
>
> "Oh," he said, "my Angel is here. I'm going to have a shower today?"
>
> "No, you get a shower on Mondays and Thursdays."
>
> "You going to get me up?"
>
> "Yes, I'll come back, but first I have to get some others up, and then I'll come back."
>
> So I came back. He took my hand and kissed it. What a compensation! What a gift! And that really makes my day.

Further out in this third circle are people that we view with distain and distrust. I suspect that every society has in groups and out groups. In 2004 Marion and I spent a month with some who belong to a large out group in

# Kindness

America—the homeless. We worked with a major Seattle homeless program. Marion spent time with some women's programs, and I worked with men's programs. The homeless definitely belong to an out group, for many in our society look down upon the homeless as irresponsible and lazy. One recent study revealed that while a majority of Americans support programs to help the homeless, they want the homeless to keep their distance.[5]

More broadly, our bitterly partisan political division in contemporary America breeds attitudes, words, and actions that demean and scorn those of opposite political persuasion. This highly polarized political atmosphere breeds not only avoidance of those from the other camp, but fosters ridicule and contemptuous words that strengthen the division. There is a great need not only for respect toward those with opposing political convictions, but also kind, charitable words and actions.

At the outermost part of this third ring are individuals from a group that we truly fear. We are suspicious of such people; with them we have our guard up. I remember being the object of deep suspicion back in 1983 when I flew from Johannesburg, South Africa to Bulawayo, Zimbabwe. At that time, South Africa was still under the apartheid policies of the white-controlled government, and through armed struggle Zimbabwe had recently shifted from white rule to black rule. As I was seeking to leave the airport in South Africa a white official eyed my passport and me with hostile distrust, and when I, a white American coming from South Africa, landed in Zimbabwe the black airport officials held me back, studied my passport carefully, and searched my luggage until my black Zimbabwean host finally arrived and quickly gained my release. Of course, in reality I was never at serious risk in either situation, because I was an American and both South Africa and Zimbabwe wanted friendly relations with the United States. Yet this gave me a taste of the vulnerability of those who must face strong suspicion.

We are understandably wary of strangers from a group that we fear, because we believe some persons from that group have been dangerous to our group. We need to be on guard for our own safety and the safety of those for whom we are responsible. Nevertheless, even with those whom we meet with fear and deep caution, Jesus calls us not merely to avoid being cruel to them, but to be good to them. "Love your enemies, do good to

---

5. Scott Clifford and Spencer Piston, "Americans Want to Help the Homeless—as Long as They Don't Get Too Close. This Explains Why," *The Washington Post*, July 14, 2017.

those who hate you, bless those who curse you, pray for those who abuse you" (Luke 6:35). This is a tall order indeed.

## Nurturing Kindness in our Caregiving

How does the kindness Jesus talks about come to reality for us in caregiving? For those of us giving care with a family member or dear friend, we may start out with a solid base of love for the person, a strong desire and commitment to care for that person, to help through this difficult time. Most of my interviews with family caregivers revealed a long-term relationship of deep regard and love for the person needing care. In nearly all cases I dealt with, whether religious or non-religious, the caregivers had a close personal relationship with the person receiving care.

Many of them also had a long history of shared religious practice that fosters kindness. As one wife of a retired pastor said:

> We get the daily devotions from the seminary, online. This is online every day, written by seminary grads and sent out to seminary grads. So they're written by lots of people we know. It's a Scripture and a devotion. We did that every day. We'd done that for years. That was a very good thing for keeping both of our moods on an even keel. Because it kept something that was very important to us in front of us. Because sometimes it was on getting rid of resentments or sometimes it was on forgiveness, sometimes on praise, charity—all the Christian virtues, and the problems as well. . . . But there were times when the mood was a little bit hard to deal with.

Another woman caring for her elderly mother commented:

> My daily devotions of reading Scripture and prayer help me center and prepare for whatever the day brings. It might be I am called by the facility once or twice a night because she is being combative. Or, it might mean making some important decisions regarding medication that we are using. The tough days are when she is so non-responsive that you are not sure she will ever be able to connect again. With God, I am able to be in the moment, pray over her (even on the days she cannot "reach back" in a tangible way, and sing hymns with her (which ironically her heart/head still remember). Mom sings hymns and children's songs to the stuffed animals she cares for like babies every day.

## Kindness

Another woman who devoted about a decade to caring for her husband said, "It's funny, because people thought I had so much patience. [laugh]. I didn't feel like I had so much patience, because there were times when it's hard to be kind."

I asked, "What did you do to restore or strengthen your patience and kindness?"

> Well, one of my kids gave me this beautiful bound book, *Jesus Calling*. And I'd read that every morning, and somedays that was just what I needed. Here is this message, as one person wrote, "Many days I felt I'd reached the end of my rope." I still need God's gift of strength to deal with the mix of emotions that come with this.
>
> And having lived here all my life, practically, I had so many friends here. And I think women are more ready than men to open up and ask for help.

A non-religious caregiver who deeply loves her mother has found that a key for her is to take time alone by going for a walk or to the gym, doing some gardening, taking a shower, listening to some soft music while focusing on her breathing. She said,

> It's so difficult, but I do find I'm more calm afterward. It's like a pressure value. Without that, you'll just explode. And I've done that. And after I've exploded, I just think, 'Why did you do that?' The guilt.

While most people I interviewed had a strong, positive relationship with the person for whom they cared, that was not true for all. An exception was a wife whose husband had had dementia for many years. I called her and asked, since they had had such a difficult relationship, why she visited him every day at the nursing home. She acknowledged that often he was not very nice to her when she visited him, yet she said, "I guess that's who I am: forgiving people. I even did *want* to go." Pausing a while, she called attention to their beautiful children. Rather than dwell on the negative aspects of their marriage, she focused on the positive fruit of the conflicted relationship with her husband.

Nevertheless, even though we caregivers may enter a caregiving relationship with a reservoir of good will toward the person and have positive, even precious memories to draw upon, there will likely be times when our kindness is sorely tested. As a daughter commented about her father's faithful care for her mother with dementia, "If someone would ask me, 'What does love look like?' I would point to Dad. His whole life, but especially in those last years, when Mom was in the care facility and not able to give back to the relationship."

Is there anything we can do to develop, strengthen, and maintain a high level of this "deeper kindness"? In general, for Christians, any practice that fosters a close relationship with Jesus Christ and the love of God will tend to form and increase this deeper kindness. The closer we are to Christ and God's love, the stronger will be our kindness toward the person for whom we give care. Yet there is no single magic way to access that divine love. So, it is not surprising that I received various answers to this interview question: "What role, if any, have your personal faith and spiritual practice played in your caregiving?"

An upper middle-aged son caring for both parents replied, "The first thing that came to mind was the consolation of intercessory prayer. . . . To this day, I really rely on that intercessory prayer for my parents, because there are such limits that we can provide them."

As noted earlier, the daughter of a woman with Alzheimer's finds renewal in her daily devotions:

> My daily devotions of reading Scripture and prayer help me center and prepare for whatever the day brings. It might be I am called by the facility once or twice in a night, because she is being combative. Or it might mean making some important decisions regarding medication that we are using. The tough days are when she is so non-responsive that you are not sure she will ever be able to connect again. With God I am able to be in the moment, pray over her (even on the days she cannot "reach back" in any tangible way), and sing hymns with her, which, ironically, her heart/head still remember. Mom sings hymns and children's songs to the stuffed animals she cares for like babies every day.
>
> When the days are tough, I am also reminded that the cross is our way through the suffering. This journey leads to restoration and resurrection. Having that hope enables me to reflect this light to my mom and those that provide care for her. It is a lovely gift, indeed.

Another middle-aged daughter caring for her mother with Alzheimer's was surprised by an unexpected blessing:

> I went through a period of being angry with God. Dad died in 2005. Mom said she was ready to go back then. There were times when I was watching her deteriorating that I started telling God that I would do a better job at being God than he did. I didn't

understand why God wasn't just taking her home. Then one day I had a client who had been a heroin and meth addict for years. She went through our treatment program and got clean and sober, and then she came to work at the facility where my mom lived.

One time this woman showed up in my office. She said, "I have to tell you something. I was helping your mom get ready for bed last night. And she put her hands on both sides of my face and said, 'You are such a sweetie.'" The woman broke down crying at that point and said, "No one in my whole life has ever called me a sweetie." I started to tear up too, and all I could think of was, "I am so sorry. I've been so short-sighted."

It is likely that there will be moments when we are unkind to the person for whom we are the primary caregiver. Even when our long-term relationship with that person has been strongly positive, on occasion, we may be irritable and short-tempered. As our level of fatigue increases, the likelihood of saying an unkind word or doing an unkind action increases. So, we also need to be kind to ourselves as caregivers by letting go of our failures and, if possible, receive the kindness of others who enable us to have time away for rest and renewal.

Whereas we may do caregiving in a strongly positive relationship with a beloved member of our family, those who do caregiving professionally must deal with a wide range of non-family people including many who are unhappy with being in a care facility. Some residents are ornery and even liable to strike out at those who attend them. Kind treatment of an unhappy, ill-tempered resident calls for prudent restraint of one's own tendency to respond in similar fashion. As one CNA said:

> I remember a nurse working with me was going to this man's room to give him his medicine. An aide was there also. Apparently, the man refused to take his medicine. The man and the nurse started to talk loud. The nurse totally lost it. Another aide was watching this from the hallway. When I went up there, this aide said, "They're arguing." I went in and suggested the nurse and aide go out of the room. The moment they lost it with this man, they should have left the room. I just held the man's hands, and he looked at me and he smiled. I said I'd sit with him.
>
> He said, "No, I want to go to my house."
>
> So I took him and we walked in the hallway. And he calmed down. So the nurse told me to give him the medicine, and I did.

I replied, "These are some of the things you say about your work as a CNA that come across to me: it's hard work, the pay is not good, and there is a lot of pressure from the supervisors and nurses. Yet you say you love some of the residents."

She answered,

> I love all the residents, even the crabby ones. Because when they're so mad, they're hilarious. Sometimes they punch you in the face, and it comes as a big surprise. That is when you have to say, "I've got to get out of the room, before I react in the same way." You learn through the years to know, really.
>
> Here is something I posted on my Facebook page: "One of the things you have to learn in life is how to remain calm. When you have it really hard, you learn lots of things. You become more than the person who started—unconfident, now confident, not shy (well, I'm still shy). But you learn to go the extra mile, more than other people do, to give the most you can do, do the best I can. I don't do it because the boss tells me. I do it because I enjoy my job. I *love* my job. It's such a hard job. Not just for me, but for everyone who has the job."

## Receiving Kindness

Our kindness as caregivers to someone in our family, a dear friend, or clients in a care facility is nurtured and sustained by receiving kindness ourselves. We cannot continue to manifest kindness to our loved one, friend, or client in need of care without being supported by the kindness of others and being kind to ourselves.

Family members and friends may rely upon the help of paid professional caregivers who come to the home or work at a care facility, but also they may look to other sources of social support. Nationally organized groups on Alzheimer's and Parkinson's provide both helpful information and the support of others in similar circumstances. As the wife of a man with Parkinson's noted, "We went to the Parkinson's support group a number of years, and that was very helpful. I believe it was particularly helpful for my husband, because you see people at various points in their progress in the illness, so to speak. So you see what is likely to happen in a year or two. That was very helpful." A retired physician caring for his wife with Alzheimer's found helpful online information on the disease from a Johns Hopkin's Medical School program.

## Kindness

Another valuable resource for family or friend caregivers is having other family members or friends who listen and support them in their caregiving. One woman, who cares for her widowed mother in a care facility, said, "My church friends have been a tremendous support. If I was traveling, they would actually set up a team of people to go visit Mom once a day, so she still had that outside support. They'd also let me vent. Let me be sad, if I'm sad. They're a safe space for me." Another woman caring for her mother has reconnected with some of her old hometown friends. "I try to keep in touch with friends here. Two of them, like me, have lost a brother. Another friend works at one of the hospitals here. It helps to keep these relationships. Some of them have gone through caregiving issues. One has a daughter who had a traumatic brain injury, so she does the majority of the caregiving for this daughter. . . . It's important to have people to talk to, to know that you're not alone."

In my own case, I look especially to our three children, who give me periodic relief. I find that after several months, I get very tired and consequently more irritable. As my fatigue increases, my ability to sleep through the night usually decreases, so my fatigue grows even more. Since our three children do not live nearby and they each have a responsible job, I must arrange well in advance with them to come for a forty-eight-hour stay with Marion, while I go away for a private retreat. Fortunately, they have been willing to help in this way. However, it means that I must plan ahead eight weeks or more. The result has been that sometimes I find myself dragging through the last couple weeks before one of them arrives. But without their support, I would be a basket case.

In addition, I find support also from some friends, especially those who are also experiencing the difficulties of being a caregiver. Although these friendships are now mostly long distance, connecting online or by phone is very valuable.

As caregivers, we are called not only to perform certain actions necessary for another's physical existence, we are also called to care for that person with kindness. This means being alert to that person's physical, emotional, and social needs and also seeking to meet those needs. At times we are likely to behave like the priest and the Levite who see a person in need, yet pass on by. Long-term caregiving inevitably brings instances of personal failure. We will be unkind to the person for whom we are caregiving. So it is also important to be kind to ourselves. By stepping away for a while from our responsibilities and gaining some perspective on our own situation, we may see our own need not only for relief and help, but also the need to be kind to our self by forgiving our self.

In our culture and in religious circles, much more attention is given to forgiveness of others than to forgiveness of self. So it is not surprising that in a study of the relationship between forgiveness of self and forgiveness of others among 364 recovering alcoholics over a two-and-a-half year period, researchers found that the participants were more forgiving of others than of themselves. The researchers also found that forgiving others had twice as strong an effect on self-forgiveness than the reverse. Nevertheless, both forms of forgiveness increased over time.[6] Since we who do caregiving over many months and even years inevitably act in unkind ways to others, we stand in need of forgiving ourselves.

---

6. A. R. Kretzman, J. R. Webb, J. M. Jester, and J. L. Harris, "Longitudinal Relationship between Forgiveness of Self and Forgiveness of Others among Individuals with Alcohol Use Disorders," *Psychology of Religion and Spirituality* (May 10, 2018), 128–37.

CHAPTER EIGHT

# Goodness

THE NEXT GREEK WORD Paul uses in describing the fruit of the Spirit in Galatians 5:22 is *agathosuna*, a noun related to the Greek adjective *agathos*, which means good. There was a long tradition of profound thought about the good in the cultures of the ancient Mediterranean world. The great Greek philosopher Plato, who lived about 428/27 to 348/47 BC, made the idea of the Good the pinnacle of his philosophy and the goal of the moral life. While there is a religious note to Plato's thought on the Good, a clearly humanistic understanding of goodness and doing good ruled with Aristotle and later Stoic philosophers, who focused on the good that we through our own understanding and moral effort ought to do.[1]

Old Testament writers had a significantly different perspective on goodness, because they focused on God as the highest good and on God's will expressed in the Old Testament law as the standard of goodness. So 1 Chronicles 16:34 teaches, "O give thanks to the Lord, for he is good." And Psalm 118:1 says, "O give thanks to the Lord, for he is good; his steadfast love endures forever!" The Old Testament prophet Micah, who lived about 737–696 BC, said the good is not just offering sacrifices. "He has told you, O mortal, what is good; and what does the Lord require of you but to do justice, and to love kindness, and to walk humbly with your God?" (Mic 6:8).

Saint Paul shares this conviction that God is the standard of goodness, but he also emphasizes that God is the source of goodness in our lives. In Romans he says, "For I know that nothing good dwells within me, that is,

---

1. Walter Grundmann, "*Agathos*," *Theological Dictionary of the New Testament* (Grand Rapids: Eerdmans, 1964), vol. 1, p. 11.

in my flesh. I can will what is right, but I cannot do it. For I do not do the good I want, but the evil I do not want is what I do" (Rom 7:18–19). Paul uses the noun, *agathosuna*, "goodness" in Galatians 5:22, as well as in three other letters. In these three other cases the New Revised Standard Version translates *agathosuna* with some variation of "good." In Romans 15:14 Paul says, "I myself feel confident about you, my brothers and sisters, that you yourselves are full of goodness [*agathosuna*]." In Ephesians 5:8–9 he says, "Live as children of light—for the fruit of the light is found in all that is good [*agathosuna*] and right and true." In 2 Thessalonians 1:11 Paul writes, "To this end we always pray for you, asking that our God will make you worthy of his call and will fulfill by his power every good resolve [*agathosuna*] and work of faith." It is odd, therefore, that in Galatians 5:22 the New Revised Standard Version translates this same word, *agathosuna*, as "generosity." Two other recent major English translations—the Revised English Bible and the New Jerusalem Bible—translate the same word in Galatians 5:22 as goodness.[2] Since "generosity" loses sight of an important Pauline insight, we will follow the more usual translation of *agathosuna* as goodness.

"Goodness" can be used in a variety of ways. When we speak of someone as a good athlete, good mechanic, good artist, or good cook, we mean they are capable at that endeavor. But being good at a particular skill does not necessarily mean one is good in a moral sense. It is well known that Babe Ruth was a very good, indeed outstanding baseball player, but he had major moral faults. In his commentary on Galatians, biblical scholar Richard Longenecker says that *agathosuna* has a range of meanings including goodness, righteousness, prosperity, and kindness.[3] When Saint Paul lists *agathosuna*, goodness, as a fruit of the Spirit, he is emphasizing that moral and spiritual goodness come from the Holy Spirit. In other words, our moral quality, our ethical well-being, and so our fulfillment as a human being comes to us as gift from God's active presence in our lives, that is, from the Holy Spirit. This can be true whether or not we as individuals acknowledge God's Spirit, although acknowledgment opens a wider door to our life.

Paul's inclusion of this broad category of goodness, *agathosuna*—so central to the ethical thinking of the dominant culture of his day—among the fruit of the Holy Spirit underscores the Christian claim that faith in

---

2. Three major commentators on Galatians also translate *agathosuna* in this passage as goodness: Hans Dieter Betz, *Galatians* (Philadelphia: Fortress, 1979); Frank J. Matera, *Galatians* (Collegeville, MN: Liturgical, 1992); and Richard N. Longenecker, *Word Biblical Commentary: Galatians* (Dallas: Word, 1990).

3. Longenecker, *Word Biblical Commentary: Galatians*, 262.

## Goodness

Jesus Christ moves a person's life toward genuine human fulfillment. This is a claim that we contemporary Christians should also make in a nuanced manner. No doubt those of us within the Christian community fall well short of being perfect models of kindness and other aspects of human goodness, yet it is helpful to call attention to the powerful presence of God's Spirit as the ultimate source of authentic human well-being.

Indeed, several of my interviews revealed signs of the Spirit's work of generating goodness in some of those who do long-term caregiving. There was the CNA whom one of her nursing home male residents referred to as "Angel"; that elderly man saw goodness in her. There was the eighty-something wife, who took care of her husband for more than ten years; she said her children all thought she had so much patience, but she did not feel patient. There was the father caring for his wife, whose daughter declared about him, "Everything he did was focused on what is best for her."

What does Paul gain by adding *agathosuna* to his fruit of the Spirit? I suggest that there are two points relevant to caregiving:

1. The subordinate point in the emphasis on goodness in caregiving is a close link to high quality care. Poor quality care, such as failing to keep a person clean, provide clean sheets and clothing, or giving the wrong medication, is to be avoided.

2. However, the main point of goodness for us is that through our difficult work of caregiving, God's Spirit is secretly working to bring forth positive moral and spiritual fruit through us and in us. Having this inner work of the Spirit affirmed by Paul is encouraging for us who tend to focus on the tedious, sometimes frustrating aspects of daily care. This emphasis on goodness as a fruit of the Spirit deepens our understanding of the grace that God has to give us who do long-term caregiving. It is a reminder that God is likely doing much more in our life and in the recipient of care than we realize.

I received such a reminder one night in March 2019. As usual I came to bed several minutes after Marion. I reached over and touched her leg. Her hand grasped mine.

I said, "Sleep good, Mrs. Hanson."
She said, "Sleep good, Mr. Hanson."
I said, "I love you."
She said, "I like it when you say that . . . I love you."

As we grip hands, I am touchingly reminded of the deep goodness in our long marriage relationship. Our marriage is indeed a great blessing.

CHAPTER NINE

# Faithfulness

WHEN WE ARE ENGAGED in caregiving for the long term as family member, friend, or professional, we have a profound and lasting need for faithfulness. The Greek word Paul uses in Galatians 5:22 is *pistis*, which in most New Testament contexts is translated simply as "faith." But here *pistis* is rightly translated as "faithfulness," in order to emphasize the ethical thrust of Paul's thought in this context. This active ethical thrust of faith deserves underscoring, because we usually understand *pistis* as primarily trust in God, a stance that is more passive, receptive to God's will. However, what Paul has in mind in Galatians 5:22 is faith as active response to God's will, so his meaning is closer to faith as obedience, the steady performance of duty.

New Testament scholar James Dunn calls special attention to this ethical dimension of faith:

> Faith in the Pauline letters is usually thought of more or less exclusively as a soteriological concept, the means through which individual and church receive the saving grace of God. The dominance of the formula "justification by faith" in discussions of Paul's theology has helped reinforce that impression. As indeed Paul's own use of the term, so heavily concentrated as it is in his own discussions of justification. In fact, however, faith is just as important in Paul as an ethical concept, as that out of which believers live. It could hardly be otherwise, since for Paul faith is the human response to all divine grace, the junction box, as it were, through which the transforming power of God flows into and through the life of individual and church.[1]

---

1. Dunn, *Theology of Paul*, 634.

It is noteworthy that in the Epistle to the Romans, which includes a classic statement of Paul's teaching of justification by faith, Paul's first use and last use of the word *faith* have a clear ethical thrust. In Romans 1:5 Paul says he has received "grace and apostleship to bring about the *obedience of faith* among all the Gentiles." And with his final use of "faith" in Romans 14 Paul addresses the differences among Christians over religious concerns about eating certain foods. Some believe they should refrain from certain foods, while other Christians believe they may eat anything. Yet those who feel free to eat anything should take care not to cause offense to the others. Paul is saying that both are making their moral judgments about food in faith. Again, faith has ethical significance.

In Paul's view, faith is absolutely fundamental to the Christian's day-to-day life. Faith is not merely having certain beliefs, holding certain things to be true. Faith for Paul is the basic stance of openness to God in both trust and obedience. James Dunn uses two metaphors to express the nature of faith as the fundamental avenue through which God's influence shapes the Christian's life and action. He says that "faith is the '*port*' through which the power of life flows" and "the *junction box*, as it were, through which the transforming power of God flows into and through the life of individual and church."[2]

"Faith" to Paul has a specifically Christian character with beliefs about God, Jesus, and human beings, which together make up a Christian understanding life. But "faith" for Paul also includes trust in the God revealed in Jesus Christ as well as obedience to this God, which is expressed in care for the well-being of others.

It is important to recognize that faith in some sense is also fundamental to absolutely every human being, whether one is religious or not. Faith is complex; it includes four main elements: belief, commitment, trust, and hope:

1. A person's faith—religious or non-religious—includes certain *beliefs*. Having a belief is holding something to be true. The beliefs that are pertinent to a person's faith are those beliefs that together make up that person's interpretation of the journey of life, beliefs that constitute that person's perspective on life and its purpose. Whether a person has a belief in God or not has an enormous impact on the nature of that person's faith. If one affirms some sort of belief in God, then one's

---

2. Dunn, *Theology of Paul*, 634, 636; italics added.

faith is also shaped profoundly by one's specific beliefs about God. For example, is God aloof or near? Is God primarily loving or judgmental?

2. Faith also includes fundamental *commitments*, what matters to a person, and centrally what matters *most*, the person's ultimate commitment. We all have many commitments; for example, to show up for work next Monday or to have lunch with a friend tomorrow. But the commitments that belong to our faith are our most basic commitments, those that underlie and take priority over lesser commitments. We prioritize our commitments all the time. For instance, we may have a commitment to meet a certain friend for lunch next Tuesday. But if a close member of our family suddenly becomes seriously ill, we cancel that lunch commitment and attend to the sick family member. Our commitment to close family members is more long-term, more fundamental. We may also have commitments to moral principles such as honesty or loyalty. It matters greatly whether we have a strong commitment to personal comfort or to care for others, to personal wealth or to generosity toward others. Our most fundamental commitments are those that belong to our faith, whether it is religious or non-religious.

3. A person's faith also includes *trust*. Trust is common in human experience, for we trust in certain people such as the best friend with whom we have shared a personal secret. We also trust a variety of organizations such as Amazon and the US Postal Service to deliver the item that we have ordered as a gift for a loved one. But the trust that belongs to our faith is our most fundamental trust, our most basic trust. On what do we rely for our fundamental meaning and security?

4. Yet another aspect of personal faith is *hope*. We all have some specific hopes. We have hopes for this or that project that engages our current energy. We have hopes for our significant personal relationships. We may have hopes about our nation's future. However, the hope that is integral to our personal faith is hope for our ultimate future. Do we look forward to some form of personal life after death? Or do we think that while death is the end of us as an individual being, some of our personal achievements may continue to have influence on others? Obviously, what we hope for is deeply influenced by our beliefs, what we hold to be true. If we deny the existence of God or some eternal ultimate reality, then belief in a personal life after death becomes unlikely.

Fundamental to every person's faith, religious or non-religious, are these four elements: belief, commitment, trust, and hope.

I asked most of those I interviewed this question: "What role, if any, have your personal faith and spiritual practice played in your caregiving?" The question usually tapped something very deep in that person's life. For instance, a man caring for his wife with Alzheimer's replied:

> I'm going to get emotional here [voice breaks]. [Faith has] had everything to do with it. Because I felt, I've had a wonderful seventy-eight or eighty years. The Lord has been very good to me. This was a part of my situation. I had life so easy, so predictable. But it's not that I had it without some work. The Lord has been there at every bend in the road. I only appreciated it in retrospect. I've seen pain going around me with people around me. Then this came along. I said, "This is my lot. The Lord is there to help me."
>
> But there is also something that came early in my life. I suspect that came from my parents: the Lord will help those who help themselves. So faith has been *clearly* . . . I'm not sure what I would have done without my faith. Because it has been rock solid . . . Through my lot in life, I've met oodles of people much smarter than me, much more gifted than I, but I made up my mind that nobody would outwork me, and nobody ever has. With my work ethic and faith, I would simply be successful in this last problem. So in a word, I couldn't be as successful in this without my faith.

A daughter caring for her mother with Alzheimer's gave this reply to my question, "What role, if any, have your personal faith and spiritual practice played in your caregiving?"

> A lot, a *whole* lot. There were days when Mom lived with us that when I'd come home from work, she'd tell me how God had spoken to her and shown her things. She would be describing beautiful colors and soothing music, and all the babies, and the many people having prayer meetings. She'd be glowing telling me about this. And I would know that she hadn't left her room all day long. As a parent, if my child was limited by a mind and body that didn't work as it should, I would most certainly take my child out on outings to show them things. I've always believed that God is, above all, a loving parent. I absolutely believe that even then God was taking my mom to heaven and showing her delightful things. She wasn't just sitting in her room all day long.

## Faithfulness

A wife, who cared for her husband with Parkinson's, said this about the role her personal faith and spiritual practice played in her caregiving: "It has been a lot through what I've been saying. The daily devotions and reading Bible stories.... Romance is great, but in the long run, kindness and patience and forgiveness are what keep a marriage going. I write that in cards to people. Extending kindness and love, not judging."

A woman caring for her mother with dementia said, "Well, I don't know how people do it without faith. That is definitely a lifeline for me. I know that I am not alone on this journey, nor is my mom alone in those times when she cannot connect with us. I know that God holds her. That's huge, just huge."

A profound feature of any caregiving relationship is how the character of that relationship reveals the caregiver's actual, lived faith. This is true whether or not the people involved even speak of their "faith." A case in point is the family in which long-term, willing caregiving of the mother has been sustained by the two adult children, who are non-religious and do not talk about their "faith." That terminology does not naturally appear in their speaking. Nevertheless, their conduct manifests their non-religious faith.

When the father died in 1998, the mother was left alone. She was seventy-eight years old and in good health. The only son, who was single and without children, gave up his job and moved back to his midwestern hometown. He thought he could get a job there, and that proved to be the case. His intention was to help his mother by maintaining the house and yard and also providing some companionship. After several years, she had a fall and thereafter needed a walker for stability. They hired a female home health aide to assist with her bathing. The daughter, who lived on the west coast with her family, regularly came for a month-long summer visit. In 2012—after about fourteen years of caregiving his mother—the son was diagnosed with cancer, which could not be surgically removed. Nonetheless, he continued to be the primary caregiver for his mother. In June 2016 when his last-ditch chemotherapy treatment failed, his sister left her husband and college senior son out west, and took up residence to care for both her brother and their mother. The three of them discussed the possibility of the mother going to a nursing home, but the mother wanted to stay in her house, and the son and daughter honored that wish. Aside from a two-and-a-half-day visit west for her son's college graduation, the daughter provided care for her brother until his death at the end of August 2016. Since then she has been the caregiver for her mother.

In view of her brother's impending death, the daughter discussed with him his final arrangements. The daughter said:

> He basically stated that he wanted the very minimum. No funeral, no wake, nothing. He also wanted to be cremated. He and I revisited the topic regarding him quite a few times.
>
> I finally convinced him to do a Celebration of Life event, which is what we did for him at the Masonic Temple. I believe he finally agreed to something like that as a "closure" event for our mom. I did have to laugh when I brought the subject up of a Celebration of Life, as his response was "Well, why bother when I'm not going to be there to celebrate?" So that's when I (along with a few of his friends) decided to do a "gathering" over at the local bar (his favorite hangout) about a block from our house. He came with his oxygen tank in tow. I called quite a few people and others passed the info by word of mouth. People were invited to come by to say "hello" or "goodbye," have a beer, talk, and visit for a few hours. Forty-some people came and went, but we had a nice turn out, and I think he was surprised by some of the people who came. My son flew in from California and was here for that as well. Although he [her brother] was pretty sick and in hospice at the time, I'm so glad we pulled that off.

After his death, the sister arranged a celebration of life at the Masonic Temple, although the family had no special connection with the Masons. She set up a memory board and a memory table with various pictures and objects recalling her brother's interests, such as his passion for the Chicago Cubs and Bears and the Green Bay Packers. She gave the eulogy. More for the sake of the mom, who attended, she had a clergyman from a local educational institution "be the emcee" and give a talk. A guitar player did a few songs, and a potluck followed. As the sister said, it was "a very low-key thing."

To repeat, *faith—any faith, religious or non-religious—has at least four basic elements: belief (holding certain things to be true), fundamental commitment, trust, and hope.* Although the mother seems to have some religious connection, neither the son nor the daughter is religious. While the son's faith and the daughter's faith are not expressly articulated, some contours of this non-religious brother's and sister's faith are evident in their behavior. For example, it is unclear what beliefs the son or daughter have about the meaning of life and the existence and nature of God. It appears that the son does not have a belief or hope for some sort of afterlife. While these three

## Faithfulness

family members have a very high level of trust in and commitment to one another, it is not clear whether the son and daughter have any belief in some greater reality. What is very clear, though, is their strong commitment to care for their mother, to make the last years of her life as good as they can be. Both the son and daughter make very significant alterations in their life, in order to help their mother through her final years. While some people do caregiving for a family member out of family pressure or guilt, both this son and daughter willingly make major changes in their own lives, in order to help their mother. Such a strong, long-term commitment is admirable.

Acting faithfully as a caregiver has somewhat different resonance depending on whether one is a family member, personal friend, or professional caregiver. Professional caregivers have the same possibility as those who have a different workplace calling—to serve God by serving other people. One may serve other people as a supermarket checkout person, a truck driver, an insurance agent, a teacher, a police officer, or a parent. Each of these roles can be understood as a divine calling, a constructive endeavor in which God calls one to serve others. So also, professional caregivers are called to serve the persons under their care.

Unlike the ordinary professional caregiving relationship, a caregiver and recipient of care from the same family bring their personal history with one another. In my case, Marion and I bring more than fifty-eight years of shared life together. Of course, from time to time each of us has disappointed the other, but we have never had a serious breach in our relationship. Since we first met, it has been impossible for either one of us to think of our own life story without including the other. The strength of that life story undergirds Marion today even though significant portions of our shared story have been chipped away from her memory by Alzheimer's disease. She still wants to kiss me often during the day, and she still snuggles up to me when we go to bed. I expect that at some point she will not want to snuggle with me, and she will not know who I am. But I hope to God that I will still know her and be by her side.

I am encouraged by the memory of a couple from our congregation who are now deceased. The wife, Flo, had Alzheimer's and was in the memory unit of a local care facility. Entering or leaving this memory unit required use of a password. Ed, the husband of many years, had Parkinson's and was some distance away in a different section of the same care facility. During the last few days of his life, three times attendants found Flo sitting by Ed's bed, stroking his cheek. Somehow on her own, Flo had found her way out of the password-controlled memory care unit to Ed's side. I intend to be by Marion's side until one of us no longer draws breath.

The question for me as the husband and caregiver for Marion is: how may I faithfully continue to carry out my caregiving of Marion in trust and obedience to God, open to God's influence day by day, hour by hour?

To begin, there is a solid moral and spiritual foundation for my caregiving of her. There is absolutely no doubt that I am called to be the primary caregiver for Marion. I do not try to run from that or think somebody else should do it. No, I am her main caregiver. That might not be true for someone else in a different situation. One may feel that a son or daughter, brother or sister at least ought to share this responsibility in a major way. But given the circumstances of our living situation in which Marion and I are three hours away from our nearest closest relative, the primary responsibility is mine. The central issue for every family member caregiver is: to what extent am I called to give care to this person? My answer is that caring for Marion is my primary task at this point in our lives. This takes priority over everything else.

Another aspect to the foundation for caregiving is motivation. One could do this out of guilt or social pressure, but to give care wholeheartedly is to do it in love for the person and in agreement with one's own faith perspective, religious or non-religious.

James Dunn says that for the apostle Paul "faith is the '*port*' through which the power of life flows." It makes sense to ask the very practical question of how one might foster faith as "the port through which the power of life flows." The religious caregivers I interviewed pointed to three basic kinds of practice that strengthened them in caregiving.

One basic spiritual practice is being an active member of a faith community or a supportive group, so that we as caregivers are not all on our own. One wife remembered with great gratitude the support of some members of their church for her husband. When I asked, "What resources or help have you found in your caregiving?" this woman said,

> The pastors, the church people. They were always very helpful when we came to church. And people were fairly frequent visitors [at the nursing home]. People outside the nursing home don't realize how important that is. How much it's appreciated, when it happens. And how dreary it gets when that doesn't happen. In that open area at the nursing home, he and two other men would be sitting there. And _____ as well as somebody else would come every Wednesday with cookies, and that was so nice. And they

## FAITHFULNESS

always talked sports. "What are the Cubs doing? What did Green Bay do?" So upbeat. It lifts your spirits. And it lifted *their* spirits too.

Another woman said that it is important "to have a church community and pastors that you feel you can call on and talk to. You just have to give yourself over to the faith that you've had all your life. You know, *it's what you do*. You live your life according to that faith. Those things that are valuable in your life, particularly, that keep you on the rails [soft laugh]."

A second common practice was finding some time to be on one's own. One caregiving wife noted that she insists on having "my own space and quiet time." She is able to manage that, because her husband generally goes to bed quite a bit earlier than she does. Another wife hired a caregiver for several hours each week, so that she could have her own personal time. For several years I have been able to go to my college office for weekday mornings, while Marion stayed at home. Since 2019 she has come with me to the library. For some months while I was in my small office, she sat in a nearby lounge chair looking at a book she has picked up from the nearby shelves, and then we have mid-morning coffee together in the union. When COVID hit in 2020 and much of the college library was off limits, she had to sit with me in my small office. Having her with me almost all the time, however, has not been a burden to me. Fortunately, we love each other very much, and we are still able to hug and kiss often.

Nonetheless, since the COVID pandemic made it impossible for me to go away every three months for a private forty-eight hour retreat while one of our kids stayed with Marion, my level of frustration increased. I did not directly attack Marion, but more frequently I burst out with a complaint such as, "Why is everything so damn hard?" Finally in September 2000 I was able to get away for a retreat in a hermitage, while our daughter stayed with Marion. But it would likely be nine months before I could do that again. So finding time alone was difficult in this special time.

A third common resource for religious caregivers is prayer and engagement with some written or recorded resources such as Scripture, devotional writings, or inspirational works. The advantage of such resources is that they can be accessed whenever one's schedule and personal habits allow. The specific forms of devotional practice differed substantially among those I interviewed. One wife caregiving for her husband with Parkinson's spoke of her, very short, in-the-moment breath prayers. Not formal and sit down and pray. But those momentary prayers. You find yourself saying, "What am I going to do now? Here? I need your help, Lord." Whisper prayers. That's what I always call them. I've never been a big formal pray-er. But a prayer whisperer—throughout the day, and sometimes [soft laugh], throughout the night. Feel supported and helped along the way.

Another wife, whose husband had Parkinson's, said she and her husband continued their long-held practice of using a daily devotional booklet that focused on a biblical text followed by a reflection and prayer. She said, "We did that every day. We'd done that for years. That was a very good thing for keeping both of our moods on an even keel, because it kept something that was very important to us in front of us." A daughter caring for her mother with Alzheimer's in a care facility said, "My daily devotions of reading Scripture and prayer helps me center and prepare for whatever the day brings."

Regular participation in some personal and corporate religious practices is essential for religious caregivers. There is no one-size-fits-all personal religious practice. To be sure, prayer is essential. But prayer practices differ significantly.

Non-religious caregivers may find comparable resources to sustain their faith. Basic also for them is communal support from family and/or friends. The non-religious daughter who supported her brother in caring for their mother for over a decade and now is caring for her alone, has found social support from her husband, old friends, and some fellow members of an exercise group. Second, she has found time to be on her own, sometimes by going upstairs in the house where her mother no longer goes. Third, she also has found strength in listening to music that calms her, and she does some meditation that quiets and centers her.

Faithfulness, the ethical dimension of faith, is a grace necessary for sustained, kind caregiving as a family member or a professional caregiver.

CHAPTER TEN

# Gentleness

WHEREAS IN CONTEMPORARY AMERICAN culture gentleness is understood primarily as a personality characteristic that is evidenced in having a soft voice and touch, in both classical Greek culture and in New Testament Christian communities, gentleness was highly regarded as a moral quality. In classical Greek culture gentleness was a mark of a high-minded person, who remained unruffled in the face of wrong treatment and did not lash out in anger. For the Greeks Socrates was a model of gentleness, for he faced his trial, wrongful conviction, and death by poison with calm dignity. The philosopher Aristotle regarded gentleness in response to wrong as the praiseworthy mean between anger and moral indifference. In the New Testament also, gentleness has important moral and spiritual significance as a mean between anger and moral indifference in response to wrong.

For Christians Jesus is the model of gentleness. In speaking of this quality, the New Testament uses the Greek adjective *praus*. The Gospel of Matthew uses *praus* three times in connection with Jesus, although each usage is given a different translation in the New Revised Standard Version. First, in the Sermon on the Mount, Matthew 5:5, Jesus says, "Blessed are the meek [*praus*], for they will inherit the earth." Second, in Matthew 11:28-30 Jesus says, "Come to me, all you that are weary and are carrying heavy burdens, and I will give you rest. Take my yoke upon you, and learn from me; for I am gentle [*praus*] and humble in heart, and you will find rest for your souls. For my yoke is easy, and my burden is light." And third, Matthew 21:5 reads, "Tell the daughter of Zion, Look, your king is coming to you, humble [*praus*], and mounted on a donkey, and on a colt, the foal of a donkey." Whereas a warrior king would ride on a horse trained for battle,

Jesus rides into Jerusalem on a domestic animal, a donkey. Jesus' gentleness is also graphically exhibited in his rejection of violence during his arrest in Gethsemane, when one of Jesus' followers struck the slave of the high priest and cut off his ear. The Gospel of Luke reports, "But Jesus said, 'No more of this!' And he touched his ear and healed him" (Luke 22:50–51).

Saint Paul shares this understanding of gentleness. In his letter to the Galatians 5:23 the Greek word translated as gentleness is the noun *prautas*. The associated adjective is *praus*, gentle. Like the great Greek philosophers, Saint Paul understands gentleness as avoiding, on the one hand, a harsh, angry response to a person's wrongdoing and, on the other hand, an apathetic, *laissez faire* response that lets any behavior go without reproach. *For Paul gentleness regards wrong action as consequential, but treats the wrongdoer with calm restraint.*

Saint Paul invokes gentleness in his dealings with the Christian community in Corinth that he founded and continued to nurture. In 1 Corinthians 4:14, 18–20 he writes,

> I am not writing this to make you ashamed, but to admonish you as my beloved children.... But some of you, thinking that I am not coming to you, have become arrogant. But I will come to you soon, if the Lord wills, and I will find out not the talk of these arrogant people but their power. For the kingdom of God depends not on talk but on power. What would you prefer? Am I to come to you with a stick, or with love in a spirit of gentleness [*prautatos*]?

And in another letter to the Corinthian Church, Paul advises dealing gently with a disruptive member of the congregation. "But if anyone has caused pain, he has caused it not to me, but to some extent—not to exaggerate it—to all of you. This punishment by the majority is enough for such a person; so now instead you should forgive and console him, so that he may not be overwhelmed by excessive sorrow. So I urge you to reaffirm your love for him" (2 Cor 2:5–8).

It is clear that Paul's understanding of gentleness is like that of the ancient Greek philosophers, who understood gentleness not merely as a psychological bent such as being soft-spoken, but as a moral quality by which one responds to someone's wrongdoing with restrained disapproval. Gentleness is the mean between anger and moral indifference. So Paul urges those in the Galatian church, "My friends, if anyone is detected in a transgression, you who have received the Spirit should restore such a one in a spirit of gentleness [*prautatos*]" (Gal 6:1).

## Gentleness

The understanding of gentleness in contemporary American culture is much more limited; it is mostly equated with personality characteristics such as soft speech and light touch in personal interactions, which are valued in family life. However, in American political and economic life, gentleness is widely viewed as a fault, and aggressively taking advantage of any wrongdoing or weakness in others is admired as a strength. Indeed, in Europe and the United States, with the recent surge of populist distrust of cultural elites and nativist mistrust of those who are culturally different, highly aggressive, combative leaders such as Donald Trump have gained support. The forceful person who rolls over opposition is widely regarded as a winner in business and public life.

A striking contrast is seen in Angela Merkel, chancellor of Germany since 2005 and leader of her party, the Christian Democratic Union (CDU) since 2000. Merkel's quite gentle leadership was strikingly evident in March 2018 in her negotiating a coalition government of her rather conservative Christian Democratic Union party with the more liberal Social Democrats. As the *Christian Science Monitor* reported: "The difficult task of negotiating a shared left-right government took six months of patient work and careful listening by Merkel. The parties had to compromise on issues such as tax cuts, immigration restrictions, and Germany's role in the European Union."[1]

The *Monitor* said that to Merkel the most important quality in life is humility, and it continued: "She often governs by remaining silent in a negotiation and then reframing a conflict of views by identifying the 'wiggle room' within each person's thinking.... In short, she draws people together by gentleness, or what might be called sweet and tender reason." Merkel herself said, "I am regarded as a permanent delayer sometimes, but I think it is essential and extremely important to take people along and really listen to them in political talks."[2] So while gentleness has moral significance today in personal relationships, it may also have positive impact in social and political affairs.

This deeper understanding sees gentleness as similar to patience in that both qualities embody a response to others that is calm and restrained. The difference is that while patience is restrained response to tiresome or annoying behavior such as repeatedly asking what day it is, the focus of

---

1. "Gentleness as a German Export, or the Secrets of Merkel's Victory," *The Christian Science Monitor*, March 19, 2018.

2. "Gentleness as a German Export."

gentleness is on restrained response to hostile, hurtful behavior such as physically hitting out or using abusive or demeaning language. In short, the biblical understanding of gentleness includes forgiveness.

Gentleness is called for again and again in caregiving, but it takes different forms depending chiefly on two factors: the recipient's medical condition and the relationship between caregiver and the recipient. Often in a caregiving situation, the recipient's medical condition affects his or her behavior. Those with some form of dementia may misinterpret events and strike out at a caregiver with harsh words or physical blows. As one daughter said of her father's care for her mother with Lewy body dementia, she "sometimes had moments of being combative" and would "treat him poorly." Because her father understood his wife's condition and loved her, he responded calmly and kindly. He was gentle with her.

Gentleness is more complicated and demanding for professional caregivers who do not have a long-term personal relationship of love with residents or other staff members. Professional caregivers are likely to encounter some individual residents and perhaps some fellow staff members who are hostile toward them. Of course, a family caregiver may have to deal at times with a loved one who is combative and hostile, but this is more common for those who do caregiving professionally and relate to multiple individuals. For instance, I spoke with a certified nursing assistant, who helps nursing home residents with healthcare needs under the supervision of a registered nurse or a licensed practical nurse. As mentioned in an earlier chapter, she said:

> There was one man at our facility. Happy was his name. I don't know his real name. He smiled all the time, but this time he wasn't smiling. I remember this nurse went to his room to give him his medicine, but she came out looking very anxious. Another nurse went in to give him the medicine and totally lost it. They started to talk loud. Another worker watched.
>
> I went up there, and this worker said, "They're arguing."
>
> I went into the room, and said, "Why don't you guys go out of the room; I'll take care of him." The moment they lost it with him, they should have left the room.
>
> I just held his hands, and he looked at me and he smiled.
>
> I said I'd sit with him.
>
> He said, "No, I want to go to my house."
>
> So I took him and we walked in the hallway. And he calmed down.
>
> The nurse said, "You'd better give him the medicine." So I did.

## Gentleness

A professional caregiver must deal with multiple needs of the residents. As noted earlier a CNA reported,

> Some who come there [to the nursing home] think they'll get better and go home. But they don't get better. Then their light just turns off. Their light just becomes dark. That's when we get closer at the nursing home. It's their loneliness. We see they need not just a worker, but someone to be close. One person there said my name was Angel. I don't really talk about that with people or my co-workers.
>
> One co-worker said, "He talks about angel did this or angel did that. Who is this angel?" I didn't say anything.
>
> This guy is blind, but he recognizes your voice and your smell. Every person has a smell. One day I went to work, and he was screaming and yelling. So I went in and took his hand and talked to him softly, "How are you doing?"
>
> Resident: "Oh, my angel is here. Am I going to have a shower today?"
>
> CNA: "No, you get your shower on Mondays and Thursdays."
>
> Resident: "You going to get me up?"
>
> CNA: "Yes, I'll come back, but first I have to get some others up, and then I'll come back."
>
> So I came back. He took my hand and kissed it. What a compensation! What a gift! And that really makes my day.

Brad: "As we've talked, what comes across to me is this: What you do is hard work, the pay is not good, and there is a lot of pressure from some supervisors and nurses. Yet you say you love some of the residents."

CNA: "I love *all* the residents, even the crabby ones. Because when they're so mad, they're hilarious. Sometimes if they punch you in the face, and it comes as so much a surprise, that's when you have to say, 'I've got to get out of the room, before I react in that situation.' You learn through the years to know, really.

"I love the residents. The best thing I have are the residents. I get to know them. And I stay because of them. Because they're so sweet. But with all of that, you learn what's the best way to handle your job. In just a few words: how to approach them. I just never had a problem with residents. Well, I did find a problem with some of the residents who were racists. They called me names. They make me do everything. They say, 'Do this or don't do that. OK, now you can leave the room.' Then afterward the nurse calls me and says you were mean to that patient. But I enjoy it a lot of the time. There are a lot of good people."

Brad: "So you're saying that there are a few stinkers among the residents, but most of them are pretty nice?"

CNA: "They might begin that way, but it's all how you approach them, treat them, and then they treat you. And over time they learn how to appreciate you. Yah, it's a hard job for that, for such low pay.

"When you have it really hard, you learn lots of things. You become more than the person who started—unconfident—now confident, not shy (well, I'm still shy). But you learn better to go the extra mile, more than other people do, to give the most you can do, do the best you can. I don't do it because the boss tells me. I do it because I enjoy my job. I *love* my job. It's such a hard job. Not just for me, but for everyone who has the job."

Of course, sometimes a professional caregiver may be unkind or make a mistake in caring for our loved one. The response of us who are family or friend should be measured, depending in part on the seriousness of their action. Since professional caregivers have human limitations and often work under stressful conditions, they are likely at times to fall short of the best care. However, a serious breach of good practice should be called out.

Gentleness in a biblical understanding is a moderate response to moral wrong, a response that is constructive for personal and social relations. Sometimes in caregiving, though, the patient's hurtful act arises from a distorted sense of reality and morality. A restrained, forgiving response by the caregiver, whether family member or professional caregiver, keeps the relationship from spiraling into combat. We who are primary caregivers may experience times in which we feel that other family members or friends let us down. Someone who had promised to help us may fail to follow through. Or a person to whom we turned for respite or a listening ear disappoints us. It may be unclear whether we had unreasonable expectations or we simply misunderstood one another. In any case, we feel let down. If we nurse our disappointment into a grudge, the relationship suffers serious harm. Dealing gently with that family member or friend in this matter is far better for us and for the relationship.

We caregivers need to be gentle not only with other people, but also with ourselves. Those of us who do caregiving for more than a short time discover that we frequently fall short of our best intentions. Sometimes we get irritable and short-tempered. We may turn a cold shoulder or say an unkind word to one needing care. If we are too strict with ourselves, we will soon crumble in despair. So we need to be gentle also with ourselves. We are frail creatures who get physically and emotionally tired. While we may be taken for granted by others or hear mostly complaints, we are needy beings who like to be appreciated for our efforts. Failing to receive gratitude, we may feel resentment. We may not *want* to feel that way; nevertheless, contrary to our best intentions, the resentment is there. So it is important to be gentle with ourselves.

Gentleness is an extremely valuable personal quality in caregiving. It is good to be gentle with the recipient of care, family members, other caregivers, and ourselves.

CHAPTER ELEVEN

# Relationships and Spiritual Practices in Caregiving

BOTH MARION AND I have found grace in caregiving mainly through two avenues: supportive personal relationships and our spiritual practices. My conversations and interviews with other caregivers indicate that most of them also find grace through these same readily accessible means.

## Finding Grace Through Supportive Personal Relationships

Marion and I receive grace through the support of caring family, friends, and professional caregivers. Most of us involved in caregiving—caregiver and recipient of care alike—have multiple personal relationships. For instance, like many others receiving care, Marion's relationships may be pictured in concentric circles of emotional connection. At the center is her most fundamental and strong emotional connection—Marion's relationship with me. Next come the relationships Marion has with our three children, Julie, Carter, and Kim. Somewhat further out from the center are Marion's relationships with her two living siblings, sister Elaine and brother Mike, and our three grandchildren. Beyond this are her daughter-in-law, son-in-law, and Marion's closest friends. Still further out is the circle of other friends and professional caregivers—Marion's physicians, nurses, and certified nursing assistants. As Marion's dementia advances, CNAs will likely fill more and more of her social interactions. My own concentric circles of emotional connection largely overlap with Marion's. Of course, at the center is my relationship with Marion. She is the dearest person to me. I expect that my relationships with the professional caregivers who care most and best for her will become increasingly dear to me as I rely more and more on their support for Marion.

## 1. Support Marion and I Give One Another

As Marion's primary caregiver, I am called to support and comfort her as she deals with the gradual decline in her mental capabilities. I have no doubt that helping her through this is now my foremost purpose in life. This is an arduous, distressing task, but I believe it is the most important task that I have ever been given.

For me the most immediate channel of grace for this responsibility has been Marion herself. Even though she has known and acknowledged from the beginning what Alzheimer's does to a person, she has not struck out in bitterness. Indeed, she herself has been a model of the qualities that Saint Paul recognizes as the fruit of the Spirit, especially kindness and gentleness. In fact, I called attention to these two characteristics a year prior to her Alzheimer's diagnosis in my tribute to Marion during a 2009 reception for her at our church, on the occasion of her seventieth birthday. I said to the group assembled:

> It's difficult to do justice to anyone's character, but in my estimation, a central feature of Marion's character is her patient kindness. This is the third quality that I wish to highlight. You may recall that in 1 Corinthians chapter 13 St. Paul expounds on the nature of *agape* love. He begins to describe love with these words, "Love is patient, love is kind." Marion is very patient and amazingly kind, much more than I am. This patient kindness is manifest in her sustained sensitivity to other people's needs, feelings, and especially their hurts. As many of you know from experience, if you're going through a difficult time, you're likely to receive a visit or an empathetic word from her.

I remarked on these qualities again later in an October 2017 email that I sent to our kids, "She is still the extremely kind, gentle woman we've known all along, but her short-term memory is weak and also some of her longer-term memories are not there for her now." In 2019, I continued to experience her patience and kindness, and was amazed that even when I was tired and very irritable she still offered me tender, supportive embraces.

As we noted earlier, kindness involves two fundamental moves: noticing another person's need and trying to meet that need. One basic form of

Marion's kindness to me has been her acceptance of my need to be intellectually active. The chief outlet this need has taken for the last fifty-plus years has been for me to leave home almost every weekday morning for my office at Luther College. At my retirement from teaching in 2000, I moved from my office in a classroom building to an office in the college library. Working in this office for twenty years of retirement, I have written three books and prepared oral presentations that have gradually decreased in number and now approach zero. Today, after almost two decades of retirement, ordinarily I still spend part of weekday mornings in my library office working on a book manuscript. Although I have generally taken Marion's acceptance of this pattern for granted, when I reflect on it, I see it as her benevolent gift. She has been kindly affirming who I am.

Marion's kindness toward me found a new expression in 2019. In February of that year we had been informed by two local occupational therapists that Marion's cognitive state now made her a risk for harm. This news fundamentally challenged my habit of leaving her home alone most weekday mornings. Our children and I began to feel our way toward appropriate arrangements for her care, while preserving some independence for me. My initial proposal was to have a professional caregiver at home with Marion for about fifteen hours a week, which would give me three hours away every weekday. Marion firmly rejected this. She finally agreed to have a CNA come each week to do some housework for two hours. My hope was that as Marion became more accustomed to having this woman in our home with her, we would be able to gradually increase that woman's hours. During this period of uncertainty, though, Marion continued kindly to affirm my desire to have some time in my college office.

Two months after this arrangement began, an additional possibility arose. One day in May 2019 Marion called me at my office and asked whether she could come to "where you are." I agreed, and quickly brought her to the college library. She selected a book from the stacks close to my office, and settled down in a comfortable chair nearby. Mid-morning we joined several other retired faculty in the college coffee shop, and then we returned to the library where she was content until we left for lunch at home. So simple. The next day I suggested we follow the same pattern and she quickly agreed. In the following weeks, except when I asked her to stay at home during the two hours when our CNA came to clean, Marion elected to come with me to the library.

The most striking expressions of Marion's kindness toward me have come when I have been grouchy. For instance, in mid-March 2019 I was getting increasingly tired and grumpy. Our son Kim was scheduled to come from California in two weeks and stay with Marion, while I would go on a retreat. My last restful retreat had been just prior to Christmas. So after almost three months, I was getting worn down. Consequently, I was having almost daily outbursts of anger. Although I tried not to direct my anger at Marion personally, she may have felt that there was a connection between my irritability and her situation. Yet she never criticized me. Her sustained response was sympathy, hugs, and kisses.

Her kindness toward me has included sustained gentleness. As we noted earlier, the classical understanding of gentleness—mild response to a moral wrong—has a deeper moral significance than the usual contemporary understanding of gentleness as being soft-spoken and mild-mannered. Marion has been gentle in both the contemporary and classical senses. When our children were young and at times needed discipline, Marion spoke with authority. They knew she was not a pushover. But she was never shrill, never out of control. By far her dominant demeanor over the years has been to be soft-spoken and mild-mannered. This has been certainly true throughout her relationships with family, friends, and coworkers. So she has been gentle in the contemporary sense of the word.

In addition, though, she has been very gentle in the classical Greek and Pauline understanding of gentleness as a measured, mild response to moral wrong. I have been the most frequent beneficiary of this. For example, one day in March 2019 I received a phone call from the man whose company was going to put down a new floor covering in our kitchen and laundry room. Two days earlier he had said his workmen would come on Thursday of that week. After that call Marion and I prepared the way by clearing out coats and other items from two closets, removing all items on the lowest shelf and floor of our pantry, piling all these items haphazardly in our living room, and then sweeping and mopping those floors. However, the next day the flooring man called to say that the job would have to be delayed for a week. To say the least, I did not welcome this news. Tired and grumpy, I stomped around, swore, and generally blew off steam, while we returned the scattered objects to their original places. It did not help that I had to explain what had happened several times to Marion. Since it is difficult for her to remember new information, multiple explanations of the same matter are to be expected. When I am reasonably rested, that is not a problem, but when I'm tired and irritable, explaining to her the same thing again and again is a challenge for me. I tried hard to avoid directing my anger at Marion, but very likely this time I did not fully succeed. Yet Marion continued to be kind to me by repeatedly offering solace.

Every day her behavior toward me reminds me of what a great blessing our marriage has been. Her reminders are primarily tactile. We hug and kiss often. During mid-afternoon tea, we sit close together and often touch. We frequently touch as we prepare for our late afternoon walk and then prepare supper. In the evening watching TV we sit close together on the family room couch, and later if she is still awake when I come to bed several minutes after her, we generally kiss, hold hands, and say, "I love you." She often snuggles up close to me for awhile.

In Christian theology, we talk about *the means of grace*, the means through which God makes known the divine love for us. Christian theology recognizes that the means of grace come in two broad forms—Word and sacrament. God's grace is conveyed through verbal means: spoken, written, and sung words. The usual way theologians think of God's Word is that it is expressed in the written form of Scripture and the oral form of speaking the Word in formal preaching or the informal testimony such as parents talking about God and praying with their children. In many ways, Marion's simple words, "I love you, Mr. Hanson," are a means of grace for me. Her words express not only her personal love for me, but also testify to God's generosity. The fact that we human beings have the potential to love one another deeply and faithfully is a wonderful, God-given attribute. For Marion and me to experience this potentiality of love actualized in our relationship with one another is a tremendous gift.

God's grace is also communicated through physical symbols called sacraments. Baptism and the Lord's Supper are the most widely recognized sacraments. In addition, though, some Christian traditions recognize certain traditionally significant physical symbols as "sacramentals." Examples of sacramentals are making the sign of the cross with one's hand, a cross of ashes on one's forehead on Ash Wednesday, and blessed palms on Palm Sunday. Some of Marion's actions have sacramental quality for me; they express both her love and God's love for me. When we are settling down in bed for the night and she snuggles up close to me, kisses my cheek, and says, "I love you, Mr. Hanson," I experience life as profoundly good. Her touch and kiss are "sacramentals" of love for me. It is humbling to realize that in turn, my touch and kiss are "sacramentals" of love for her.

Although none of the caregivers I interviewed *explicitly* said in their original interview that the loved one for whom they cared had been or is a mediator of grace for them, later by email I asked two spousal caregivers whether they also had experienced the flow of grace from care recipient to caregiver. I wrote to both of them:

> As I have reflected more and more on caregiving one's spouse, it has occurred to me that while I as caregiver can be a "means of grace" for Marion (in other words, an avenue for God's grace, kindness, and love to shine through), it is also true that Marion has been and is a "means of grace" for me—that God's grace, kindness, and love shine through her to me.
>
> I'm wondering whether that thought connects with anything in your own experience of caregiving your spouse.

I promptly received this response from one of them:

> Yes, it absolutely does, Brad. In all the long years of living with Parkinson's, I believe he was given extra measures of grace in order to remind me of that gift. I surely didn't recognize those gifts always, but in his steady and uncomplaining manner, I was the recipient of that grace without a doubt.

A while later the other woman told me in person how grace had blessed her relationship with her husband. It began already in how he treated her with such kindness and respect during their several years of courtship and continued all the way into his years with Parkinson's at home and in a nursing home.

In addition, I think the reality of grace active on both sides of the caregiving relationship was *implicit* in the testimony of most other family caregivers I interviewed. Not only did these caregivers mediate grace to the loved one for whom they cared, but in nearly all cases the flow of grace at times had moved also from care recipient to caregiver. If I had thought to ask all of them explicitly whether they as caregivers received grace through their care recipient, I believe nearly all would have responded in the affirmative.

## 2. Support from Other Family Members

Marion and I are very fortunate to have the support of our three children. Especially vital for me personally are the times when one of our kids stays with Marion while I am away on a private retreats. Another significant part of their assistance comes when we are faced with a major decision about Marion's care. It is a great help to know that I do not face those decisions alone. Our daughter Julie's presence at Marion's important medical appointments has been immensely valuable by adding another perspective on what is best for Marion. Julie communicates quite frequently with me, checking on how we're doing and conversing with me about current issues in caregiving Marion. I'm thankful that she does not always ratify my interpretation of events or proposal for care, but sometimes disagrees with me and suggests another way to proceed. Taken all together, our adult children's concern and commitment to the welfare of Marion and me surround us with the sustaining comfort of their love, their wisdom, and their practical assistance.

Both Marion and I have long and deep emotional connections with our three adult children. While Marion now needs to be reminded of the identity of nearly every one of her old friends, she still has emotional connections with our daughter and two sons. It is to these three persons that I have turned to stay with Marion while I go away for deep rest on my periodic retreats. It is also to them that we report on major medical appointments, as in the following email exchanges.

*Brad to Julie, Carter, and Kim, February 27, 2019*

> This is my report on our visit at the Mayo Clinic in Rochester last Friday. Julie accompanied Mom and me as we visited with a nurse practitioner.
>
> When I called Mayo for an appointment a while back, I asked that we meet with a female neurologist. I did this because, during our last visit there several years ago, the male neurologist looked only at me when he spoke, as though Mom were not really present. I asked him to speak to both of us then, but I figure that not looking directly at the person with dementia is probably his usual practice. Since I thought a woman might be better at this, I asked for a female. Since Mayo had no female neurologist, I got an appointment with a female nurse practitioner in that department. It turned out very well. As Julie commented after the appointment, an advantage is that a nurse practitioner is able to spend more time with patients. As it turned out, she had also grown up in Decorah.
>
> My chief concern coming into the meeting was to learn more about how to handle the delusions Mom has been having during

the last several weeks. The main takeaway on this for me was that we're doing about as well as can be expected. The nurse practitioner said Mom is doing very well getting regular vigorous exercise. As you know, we generally walk two miles a day or do some vigorous work outside such as Mom shoveling snow off our deck and often much of our sidewalk. The woman said there was no reason to take a medication for the delusions, since the principal medication for this is a chemical that the body naturally produces with active exercise.

One striking, but I suppose not unexpected, incident came toward the end of our visit when the nurse practitioner used a routine memory drill in which she gave Mom three words and said that after a while she would ask Mom to recall those words. Several minutes later, when asked for the words, Mom had no idea whatsoever.

I'm very glad that Julie accompanied us, because she raised some issues that I would have overlooked. So Julie, please give your thoughts on the visit.

Love,

Dad


*Julie to Brad, Carter, and Kim, March 1, 2019*

Hi all,

Thank you, Dad, for sending this report. I was also glad that I could meet you there. I have a few things to add, as well as a clarification regarding the medication.

The nurse practitioner said that exercise can produce the same effects as Aricept, which is the first Alzheimer's drug that came out. Taking Aricept on top of the exercise could have additional subtle effects in terms of treating symptoms of dementia but she didn't think it would make a big difference. Anti-psychotics would be used to treat the delusions. Since Mom isn't having delusions that frequently and doesn't get fixated on whatever the current mistaken belief is, the nurse practitioner didn't recommend starting an anti-psychotic at this time. If the delusions become more frequent and/or she keeps fixating on them, then we would need to reconsider.

The nurse practitioner thought we were right to be concerned about Mom being home alone. Since it turns out that there isn't an adult day care program in Decorah, we need to look at other options. There are adult day care programs in Waukon and another town nearby. There's a van from one of those programs that picks up people some miles outside of Decorah and takes them to the program. Another option is finding volunteers or paid home health care aides to come to the house and be with Mom. Dad, one of my colleagues suggested looking for students through the college who are looking for part-time work. Nursing or social work students might be particularly good. Mary Jane [our son Carter's mother-in-law] has also offered to spend time with Mom. Dad said he knows he'll need to stop going to the office or reduce the time he spends there. I think it's important to make sure, for Dad's mental health, that he is able to get at least some time away during the week.

The nurse practitioner also agreed it's a good thing that Mom and Dad are on waiting lists for the assisted living places, since something unexpected could happen to either one of them and it would become necessary to move.

I was also really struck by the memory test. Mom didn't know the year, the day, where she was, or what her home address is. She did a little better with repeating numbers, but didn't even attempt repeating the four words even right after the nurse practitioner said them. Mom just said she couldn't do it.

The nurse practitioner also recommended yearly visits to Mayo (it had been five or six years since the last time she was there.) Dad, I know that you don't feel there's much use to going annually because there isn't much they can do, but I think there's value in having her evaluated on a regular basis and talking about options given whatever she is currently experiencing.

Dad, please let us know what we can do to help you and Mom other than coming to stay with Mom when you take your weekend retreats. Being far away, it's difficult to know what is most useful to you.

Love to you all,

Julie

Marion's personal connection with family members to a considerable extent is inversely related to their physical distance from her. The fact that Marion feels emotionally closest to me is correlated with the fact that I live in the same house with her day in and day out. Marion's feeling of connection with each of our three children is also correlated with their physical

RELATIONSHIPS AND SPIRITUAL PRACTICES IN CAREGIVING

distance from her. In part because our daughter Julie lives the closest of our children, she is able to be present with Marion more often than our sons. Our son Carter lives 370 miles away, and our son Kim lives 1,600 miles from Decorah, so their presence with Marion requires more planning and expense. Of course, physical distance alone does not determine the depth of a personal relationship, but distance certainly affects the ability to be personally present.

### 3. Marion also Receives Grace through the Support of Caring Friends

In addition to the support Marion and I give each other and the support we receive from our family members, Marion also receives support from caring friends. One major change that comes with dementia is increased social isolation. A person with advancing dementia gradually loses the ability to interact socially with others. To carry on a good conversation with an old friend or family member requires remembering that person's identity and interests as well as some past shared experiences and anticipated experiences. As the person with dementia gradually loses those memories, the basis for conversation is eroded. So Marion's dementia eventually led us to drop out of the monthly game group of four couples that we had enjoyed for over forty years. This shrinking of social interaction makes the continued connection and support of loyal family and friends especially valuable.

Marion's continued involvement in her weekly afternoon coffee group—the Menders—has been made possible by the generous help of other women in the group. Doris regularly notifies me about their upcoming gathering and usually gives Marion a ride; if Doris is unable to do it, someone else in the group steps up. Another Menders member who cared several years for her husband told me that she didn't know what she would do without Menders. "Those women are not there to gossip, but to support one another." Even with COVID Menders have regularly met outside and physically distanced until cold weather ended that. During the colder months the group meets together virtually, but Marion is no longer able to participate in that medium. In addition to receiving help in getting to the outside meetings of Mender's, Marion's participation in her contemplative church women's group—Mary Circle—was aided by other members of the group, who have alerted her to meetings and provided transportation.

## 4. My Mixed Experience of Receiving Grace through Friends

While I have also benefited from the support of friends, especially those who are also caregivers, my experience in this respect is mixed. The reality is that my face-to-face support from close male friends has been significantly eroded as I have grown older. Especially significant losses were the deaths of two men who were open to regular deep personal sharing with me—Bernie, who died in 2001, and Paul, who died in 2017. In their retirement years these men lived in Decorah, and I met each man regularly for morning coffee or lunch. Not only did we discuss current events, but we also shared what was going on in our life. Currently I have no close male friend nearby with whom I can frequently talk in depth.

Although I no longer have a close friend living nearby, I have received much valued support from two old college friends who live far away from me, especially from C, whose wife also suffered from Alzheimer's disease. On February 22, 2019 C reported that his wife had fallen and broken a vertebra in her back.

I responded to C expressing regret, and then added:

> Just this moment, my office phone rang, and it was Marion. She said she feels as though I don't want to have anything to do with her, and would I come home. I reassured her that I love her, and I said I'd come home. So I'm going. I don't know where her feeling about that comes from except from the Alzheimer's.
>
> Well, my phone just rang again, and it was Marion saying that she now knows that everything is OK, and I don't need to come home at this very moment. That was an extremely quick turnaround—all in about two minutes. But I suppose it reveals the fragility of her emotional states. We are always very lovey dovey, so this break in her sense of my loving her comes as a big surprise. In any event, C, stay in touch about how things are going with [your wife] and you.
>
> Brad

At this point, R, another old college friend, expressed support and said, "I cried when I read your message, Brad."

I responded:

R,

I want to thank you for your message to me. What struck me most were these words of yours: "I cried when I read your message, Brad." It touched me deeply to know that I am not alone in this situation. Marion and I are very fortunate in that our three adult kids are all supportive, but it is also very comforting to know that I have an old friend who feels some of my sorrow. Thank you for your kindness.

What a long way we have come. Back when we were in college, we men would never have said anything like that to one another. Indeed, for our adult life we would have avoided such expressions of caring to another adult man. Now in our old age, I am glad to thank you for your kind words. We both have grown some over the years.

Brad

*Brad to C, April 22, 2019*

How are things going with you and [your wife], especially on how you're dealing with her needing someone nearby all the time? I'm personally engaged with this same issue with Marion. She has not had an accident, but a recent exam by two local occupational therapists resulted in their recommendation that she not be left alone. Marion is extremely resistant to having some outside person with her for many hours, and I can appreciate her feelings. Part of my reservations about leaping into so much professional help is that Marion is quite trim and nimble. We either walk two miles a day or we do outside work around the house.

We've decided to start with a home care worker just two hours a week—to vacuum, dust, etc.—we've had a person doing this for about a year now, but the new person is a CNA. I'm hoping that as Marion becomes accustomed to this woman, we can gradually increase her hours up to 15 to 20 per week. I think it's important for me to get time in my college office; that keeps me somewhat balanced.

At any rate, I'd like to know how you're handling things.
All the best,

Brad

## Finding Grace in Caregiving

*C to Brad, April 22, 2019*

Yo Brad—With the fall on 2/20, [my wife] and I entered the next phase of the journey: she could never be left alone, and by alone I mean she really needs someone at her side/in the room all the time. The falls were diagnosed as simply resulting from an over-medicated high blood pressure. She is now on no BP meds with pressures running a little higher than we'd like, but that won't kill her ... continued falling will.

A couple[of] friends recommended independent home care persons, and they have worked out quite well. They come at 10 a.m. and leave at 4. They bathe, dress, clothe, assist potty needs, and literally are with her all the time they are there. They do no cooking or housework. When I'm home during their work day, it's surprising how much more at ease I am. People kept telling me I should be getting some help, but I continued thinking, "Well, I can do this by my lonesome." One can, but it will eventually WEAR YOU OUT—and remember, if something happens to you, both of you are in big trouble. Hope this helps, Brad, and you know you can email or call me anytime.

Later, C

*C emailed again, about two weeks later*

Couple thoughts here, Brad. I think my situation is a little further down the road as regards care than yours. [My wife] could not live by herself and after the fall we've moved to the next stop down that road: she cannot be left alone and in a good way that pushed me to get someone to be here—six hours, six to seven days a week is about right. Were it not for me and the caregivers, she'd have to be in a "skilled nursing unit" ... the new moniker of what we called the old nursing home. Not only is [my wife] getting her care at about half the cost a nursing home would charge, but she's being housed in her own house and not in a bedroom at the facility; further, the care is much more personal, and the meals are far better.

The next phase, if it ever comes to that, is when [my wife] no longer knows who I am, and more importantly, becomes incontinent. I actually help her now after she's at stool with the "clean-up" which she can't do ... and I'm willing to continue to do that.

One last point. Even when I'm home and the helpers are here too, I feel much less stressed because I don't have to be with her minute-to-minute. I've gotten off to Bible School the last two

Wednesday mornings at 8, and then went fishing. So, I'm beginning to get my life back.

Later, C


*Brad to C, May 29, 2019*

C,

The last time I wrote you, I expressed satisfaction that Marion apparently had accepted the presence of our home care worker in our home. Well, there is a new turn in the saga. Today Marion said she did not want this person to be in our house. I tried to reason with her by pointing out that getting outside help is part of what happens when we get old, but this is a deep emotional issue with her.

Then Marion suggested that she come with me to the Luther College library. I said that would be fine. However, she was torn. She cried as she said she felt like she was causing a problem for me and would interfere with my work. I hugged her and reminded her that she could do what she has done several times before—sit a short distance from my office door and read a book that she has chosen. She still considered the matter a few minutes before choosing to come with me. I stuck a note for Sharon [our cleaning lady] on our unlocked front door, and we left for the library. At this moment Marion is looking over books in a history section near her seat. In a half hour or so, we'll go for coffee in the college union.

Brad


*C to Brad, May 30, 2019*

Morn'n Brad,

[My wife] has said she doesn't like either of the care givers we have that well, but my retort to her is that I NEED them and without them I couldn't keep her at home. Blunt, but the facts. I think [my wife] is a lot further down the road than Marion: she does not consider this her home and she frequently states she wants "to go home" which I think has some deep and foreboding existential elements. She's never located that place to me. Point here is I think Marion still considers your home, her home too. But Marion, as I've often talked to [my wife] about, needs to know we need our time for the health and happiness of everyone ... without making them feel guilty about their illness, which is a very tough needle to thread I know.

Day by day, trying to do our best. I envy your being able to still walk together for a cup at the Union. Later. C.

*C to Brad, June 21, 2019*

> Things steady here. Oh, at our last neurology office visit a couple weeks ago, the neurologist suggested we consider putting [my wife] under hospice. No, she said she didn't feel my wife had six months to live, but thought we would benefit from the services offered. Long story short, did just that last week. At present and the foreseeable future this means for us—weekly nursing visits, one to three times a week a certified nurse's aide will come to the house and bathe her (with the home care person I already have six hours/day/five to seven days per week), and "respite care." This means up to once a month [my wife] could be admitted to their facility for five days and I can do whatever I wish as "respite care." The last week in August [my wife] will go to Hospice House (the caregiver working for us will spend six hours each day with my wife as she now does in our home), and I'll be going to NC fishing! A wonderful service all covered completely by Medicare. Other services like nutrition help, etc. also available. Will keep you posted on that, but am really looking forward to returning back a bit to my old life. Later. C

Being able to connect with these two old friends, especially with C whose wife also has Alzheimer's, is a great comfort and support for me. I have definitely felt grace at work through our communication with one another. Nevertheless, the great physical distance between us limits all of our communication to email or phone. Until COVID shut down long-distance travel, this reality made the annual two-week Decorah visit of my friend George especially helpful. Sitting face-to-face talking over an extended lunch with this old friend was a precious gift. It was comforting and encouraging to talk openly with another elderly man.

I think male caregivers are particularly vulnerable to social isolation, because as a gender we are less willing and able to engage in deep personal sharing, especially with another man. Ask most men about recent political or sports events, and they will gladly express an opinion. But ask most men how they *feel* about the ongoing decline of their loved one, and they will probably mumble a generalization and then change the subject. If we men share our inner thoughts and feelings with anyone, we are most likely to do that with our wife or another woman. So when our wife is no longer able to share on a deep level, we are especially bereft. Deep personal sharing among men is much less common. I suspect that intimate sharing among women is also not an everyday experience, but on the whole, women are better at it than we men. Of course, women caregivers also may suffer the loss of their best friend and closest confidant, but generally women start with a wider circle of good friends. So in a long-term caregiving situation, women caregivers generally have more social support than men. As a woman in Marion's Menders group said to me, "These women are not there to gossip, but to support one another. I don't know what I'd do without Menders."

### 5. Support from Professional Caregivers

Until early 2019 the relationships that Marion and I had with her professional caregivers were mostly positive, although these relationships were very short-term or, in the case of her general practice doctor, limited to occasional appointments. Then we turned a corner in this regard as we began to rely on a home health care worker. My hope is that Marion's relationship with Sharon, our first CNA home health care worker, will grow into a strong supportive relationship, and there are signs that Marion likes Sharon. Since CNAs will most likely take over more and more of Marion's care as her Alzheimer's advances, I see it as part of my care for Marion to respect, encourage, and frequently thank those professionals who manifest quality care for her.

## Finding Grace through Personal Spiritual Practices

In addition to personal relationships as an extremely valuable source of support in caregiving, the second main channel through which Marion and I experience God's grace has been our spiritual practices. Marion has been especially nurtured through participation in the worship life and fellowship of our Christian congregation, her contemplative small group (Mary Circle), and her personal prayer practice. Marion is no longer able to tell me much about her experience of corporate worship but the fact that she continues willingly to participate in this corporate experience, chant the liturgy, and sing the hymns suggests that it is still meaningful for her. On those Sundays when I did not have choir, we picked up Marion's longtime friend Ag at her assisted living facility, and Ag sat next to Marion during worship.

However, the after-worship social experience of talking with others over coffee varies greatly in significance for Marion. Most energizing for her is when we are able to sit with a woman with whom she still feels a close connection. Marion lights up when she is able to sit with Ag, Ruth, or the daughter of an old friend. Rather surprising to me is the development of Marion's rather close relationship with Jane, who is a new friend that joined our congregation within the last few years. Before worship Jane consistently greets Marion with a warm embrace and monthly gives her a ride to Mary Circle. I was pleasantly surprised recently right after worship when on her own Marion went across the sanctuary to greet Jane. Since the number of people Marion feels close to has shrunk so much, more often than not she feels little connection with others sitting at our table during the coffee time after worship. That is part of the harsh reality of dementia.

In addition to corporate worship with our congregation, until COVID shut it down Marion continued to participate in Mary Circle, the women's contemplative prayer group that she initiated more than twenty years earlier, even though she no longer could take a leadership role and the composition of the group has changed somewhat. Although Marion was unable to tell me much about her current experience of Mary Circle, with the assistance of Jane, who reminded us of the meetings and gave her a ride, Marion persisted in going.

Although Marion is now unable to describe to me her personal prayer practice, there are indications that she no longer can continue her long time use of *lectio divina*, an ancient Christian prayer practice of letting God speak through a biblical word or phrase by reading or calling to mind the word or phrase, and listening for what God might say through it. The primary indication that she has discontinued this form of prayer in some rudimentary way is that she no longer keeps her Bible right next to the easy chair in our study. But this practice sustained her since her retirement in 1996. She would sit in that chair each morning after breakfast, and prayerfully reflect on a passage of Scripture. For many years when walking alone, she would also prayerfully listen to a portion of Scripture that came to mind. While Marion is no longer able to sustain reflective prayer, occasional impromptu

## Relationships and Spiritual Practices in Caregiving

comments from her such as "Thank you, God," lead me think she still has some awareness of God's presence in her life.

The spiritual practices that have been most meaningful for me personally have been three—sustained participation in the worship life and fellowship of our congregation, the habit of daily meditation, and periodic retreats.

1. The most mundane of my own spiritual practice has been sustained participation in the life of our congregation. Attending regular worship services at Good Shepherd Lutheran Church keeps me in touch with the Christian message and its gracious relevance to my own concrete situation. An added benefit is that this is a spiritual practice that Marion and I share together. While corporate worship helps sustain me with my personal struggles, it also tends to lift my gaze to consider the needs not only of Marion, but of others. Sometimes that need is visible in another person at worship with us; other times the need of people far away is called to our attention. Until COVID came along, especially valuable for me was my participation in our congregation's senior choir, whose director is a very talented music professor and composer. Somewhat reluctantly, Marion initially stayed home alone during my mid-week evening choir practice, but in the fall she frequently came with me and listened to practice. She willingly came early with me Sunday mornings for choir warmup.

2. In addition to participation in the life and fellowship of our congregation, a spiritual practice vital to me has been daily meditation. My core prayer practice for about forty years now has been the Jesus Prayer. Nearly every morning I devote twenty minutes to mentally repeating "Lord Jesus Christ, have mercy on me." As I do this, I normally sit in our study facing a large icon of Jesus. Of course, my mind wanders . . . *a lot*, but I keep coming back to the Jesus Prayer. A huge strength of regular Jesus Prayer practice is that often, here and there during the day and night, the prayer comes to mind of itself, especially when I am alone. It would happen often when I walk alone from our car to the college library, from the library to the union for mid-morning coffee, from our car into the supermarket, or in our neighborhood. Also the Jesus Prayer would often come when I was sitting alone in my office. The sense of God's immediate presence that the Jesus Prayer gives me is immensely life-giving. It is an incredible gift that occasionally

makes tears come to my eyes. The prayer keeps me solidly grounded and undergirds my relationship with Marion. I know that I am not alone in caregiving her; Christ is with me.

3. The third spiritual practice that has been very helpful for me has been periodic private retreats. This too has been a long-term practice of mine, one that began in the mid-seventies. My custom for the last twenty years has been to do a forty-eight-hour unstructured retreat in which I spend most of my time sitting quietly and looking out a window at nearby trees, squirrels, and birds. I welcome falling asleep in a recliner. In the afternoon I take a long, leisurely walk, and I prepare my own simple meals. Of course, I do the Jesus Prayer for about twenty minutes every morning, and the prayer often comes to me on its own at other times as I sit or walk. I find these retreats very restorative. I return home glad to see Marion and grateful to one of our kids for staying with her.

   A change that first came about in connection with my personal retreat in March 2019 was that the prospect of my leaving for retreat caused strong feelings of insecurity in Marion. Many times prior to my departure she asked me about my "going away" and wanted to know exactly when I would return. Would I be back in time on Sunday to go to church with her? Repeatedly, I told her that I thought I would return in time Sunday morning to join her midway through the worship service. In spite of the distress that Marion now feels about my leaving on retreat, I am not tempted to give up this practice, because I am convinced the retreats keep me physically, emotionally, and spiritually fit for sustained caregiving.

## Grace for Our Caregiving

The key for us caregivers to sustain kind long-term caregiving is having a patient, kind heart. No doubt there are powerful forces that pull us toward resentment, anger, and despair, chief among them physical and mental fatigue. If we go too long without refortifying our heart, we are likely to be overcome by those negative forces.

To caregivers and everyone else, the Christian message promises both forgiveness and renewal, for which the theological terms are justification and sanctification respectively. Whereas justification brings God's full forgiveness, sanctification or renewal is always partial and incomplete in this life. Extensive experience in caregiving is not required to realize that the Spirit's work of transforming grace that produces fruit of the Spirit such as love, joy, patience, and kindness are at best manifest in our life only partially and intermittently. There are times when we fail dismally to be a good caregiver. Hence it is vital to keep in mind Paul's other basic dimension of grace—justification, forgiveness. God's acceptance of us as we acknowledge our falling short is the essential companion to the call to love those for whom we are a caregiver.

Caregiving is a difficult but extremely valuable ministry. It is well to remember that it is a *ministry*, that is, a form of service. We caregivers serve not only the person or persons for whom we directly care, but often we also serve their family members. Those who do caregiving as their employment may take satisfaction and pride in having a dual ministry of serving both their patients and the family members of their patients. In those cases when professional care workers see that a patient has little or no support from family, their attentiveness as a professional is especially critical. Given the importance of good professional care, it is appropriate and, indeed, prudent for family members to express gratitude to an attentive care worker. Those of us who are caregivers for a family member are also called by God to serve in this ministry. In my own case, I not only serve my wife, Marion, but also our three children, who otherwise would be directly responsible for their mother's care. To be honest, I do not ordinarily think of my caregiving as also serving my daughter and two sons, but that definitely is part of the total picture. While caregiving is a difficult, mostly mundane, and tedious ministry, it is also a much needed and highly valuable ministry. Thanks be to God for the grace that can enable us to carry out this ministry with patience and kindness.

www.ingramcontent.com/pod-product-compliance
Lightning Source LLC
Chambersburg PA
CBHW030859170426
43193CB00009BA/672